Charles Nicolle International Conferences in Paediatrics
Colloques Charles Nicolle de pédiatrie

Recent Advances in General Paediatrics

Progrès récents en pédiatrie générale

Eric Mallet

Richard Medeiros

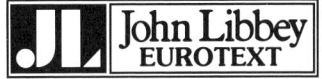

ISBN 978-2-7420-0707-3

Éditions John Libbey Eurotext
127, avenue de la République
92120 Montrouge, France
Tél. : 01 46 73 06 60
e-mail : contact@jle.com
http://www.jle.com

John Libbey Eurotext Limited
42-46 High Street
Esher
KT109QY
United Kingdom

© John Libbey Eurotext, 2008

Il est interdit de reproduire intégralement ou partiellement le présent ouvrage sans autorisation de l'éditeur ou du Centre Français d'Exploitation du Droit de Copie (CFC), 20, rue des Grands-Augustins, 75006 Paris.
It is prohibited to reproduce this work or any part of it without authorisation of the publisher or of the Centre Français d'Exploitation du Droit de Copie (CFC), 20, rue des Grands-Augustins, 75006 Paris, France.

Les coordinateurs
The editors

Eric Mallet. Chef du département de Pédiatrie, CHU de Rouen – Hôpital Charles Nicolle, Rouen, France.

Richard Medeiros. Rédacteur médical, CHU de Rouen – Hôpital Charles Nicolle, Rouen, France.

Les auteurs
The authors

Samy Cadranel. Service de Gastroentérologie, Hôpital Universitaire des Enfants Reine Fabiola, Université Libre de Bruxelles, Bruxelles, Belgique.

Olivier Dulac. Service de Neuropédiatrie, Hôpital Necker-Enfants Malades, Paris, France.

Michèle Garabédian. Inserm U561, Hôpital Saint-Vincent-de-Paul, Paris, France.

Jean-Pierre Guignard. Unité de Néphrologie, Service de Pédiatrie, CHU Vaudois, Lausanne, Suisse.

Philippe Jeammet. Service de Psychiatrie de l'adolescent et du jeune adulte, Institut Mutualiste Montsouris, Paris, France.

Hugo Lagercrantz. Karolinska Institute, Hôpital pour Enfants Astrid Lindgren, Stockholm, Suède.

Stanley Plotkin. Université de Pennsylvanie, Philadelphie, PA, USA et Sanofi Pasteur, Lyon, France.

Jean-Marie Saudubray. Centre de référence des Maladies Héréditaires du Métabolisme, Hôpital Necker-Enfants Malades, Paris, France.

Martin O. Savage. Department of Paediatric Endocrinology, Barts and London School of Medicine, London, United Kingdom.

Pierre Scheinmann. Hôpital Necker-Enfants Malades, Paris, France.

Yvan Vandenplas. Clinique Pédiatrique, Academisch Ziekenhuis Kinderen, Vrije Universiteit Brussel, Bruxelles, Belgique.

Avec l'aide de :
With the participation of:
Catherine Faber. Médecine et Enfance.
Hélène Collignon. Médecine et Enfance.

Préface

Le pédiatre d'aujourd'hui, comme tous les médecins d'ailleurs, est confronté à une nécessité vitale et inhérente à sa profession : acquérir constamment un savoir médical de haut niveau, extrêmement précis et ce, pour chacun des domaines qui le concerne. Comme pour rendre sa tâche encore plus ardue, il fait face à un nombre sans cesse croissant de revues et d'ouvrages spécialisés.

L'objectif du premier volume de *Progrès récents en pédiatrie générale* est de présenter des articles clés qui ont été rédigés par des spécialistes internationaux exclusivement pour cette série d'ouvrages. Les praticiens francophones ont aussi à leur disposition un résumé des différents ateliers qui se sont tenus lors du Colloque International de Charles Nicolle en 2006.

L'ouvrage issu du Colloque International est l'œuvre d'Eric Mallet, chef du département de Pédiatrie de l'hôpital universitaire Charles Nicolle de Rouen et de Richard Medeiros, rédacteur médical de l'hôpital

Ce volume est le premier de la collection des *Progrès récents* : il est en hommage à Charles Nicolle (1866-1936), prix Nobel de médecine pour ses recherches sur le typhus épidémique. Le second volume de la série est prévu pour 2009 et s'intéressera au domaine de l'urologie.

Remerciements

Les auteurs remercient Monsieur Christian Paire, Directeur général du CHU-Hôpitaux de Rouen, Monsieur Christian Thuillez, Doyen de la faculté de médecine et pharmacie de Rouen, Monsieur le Professeur Eric Bercoff, Président de la commission médicale d'établissement, ainsi que Monsieur Philippe Delorme, Directeur des relations internationales, pour leur soutien aux Colloques Charles Nicolle de Pédiatrie.

De même, les auteurs sont reconnaissants à Madame Muriel Clech pour son excellente assistance technique ainsi qu'à Monsieur Gilbert Surais, pour la reprographie du document, et tout particulièrement Monsieur Gilles Cahn, Directeur des Éditions John Libbey.

Foreword

The modern paediatrician is confronted, like all doctors, with the absolute necessity of acquiring a high level of specific medical knowledge concerning each subspecialty. The amount of specialised journals and text books are constantly increasing. The aim of the first volume "*Recent Advances in General Paediatrics*" is to present practical key articles written by international specialists expressly for this series. For French speaking physicians there is also a summary of the various Charles Nicolle International Workshops which were held in 2006.

The Editors and organisers of the International Workshop series are Eric Mallet, Head of the Paediatric Department at Rouen University Hospital-Charles Nicolle and Richard Medeiros, Rouen University Hospital Medical Editor.

This first volume in the *Recent Advances* series is dedicated to the memory of Charles Nicolle (1866-1936), Nobel prize laureate in Medicine for his research on epidemic typhus. The second volume of *Recent Advances* series is scheduled for 2009 in the field of Urology.

Sommaire

Les progrès récents en gastroentérologie
Samy CADRANEL 1

Les progrès récents en épileptologie
Olivier DULAC 9

Les progrès récents dans le métabolisme osseux
et phosphocalcique chez l'enfant
Michèle GARABÉDIAN 15

Développements récents en néphrologie pédiatrique
Jean-Pierre GUIGNARD 23

Développements récents en pédopsychiatrie
Philippe JEAMMET 33

Les progrès récents en néonatalogie
Hugo LAGERCRANTZ 45

Présent et futur en vaccinologie
Stanley PLOTKIN 51

Les progrès récents dans les maladies héréditaires du métabolisme
Jean-Marie SAUDUBRAY 57

Progrès en endocrinologie pédiatrique 2001-2006
Martin O. SAVAGE 63

Nouveautés en pneumologie-allergologie pédiatrique
Pierre SCHEINMANN, Rola ABOU TAAM, Jacques de BLIC,
Muriel Le BOURGEOIS, Chantal KARILA 67

Les progrès récents en nutrition
Yvan VANDENPLAS 77

Contents

Recent Advances in Paediatric Gastroenterology
Samy CADRANEL 87

Progress in Paediatric Epilepsy: 2001-2006
Olivier DULAC 103

Calcium, Phosphorus, and Metabolic Bone Diseases in Children:
What has Changed over the Past Five Years
Michèle GARABÉDIAN 119

Recent Advances in Paediatric Nephrology
Jean-Pierre GUIGNARD, *Lesley* REES 131

Recent Progress in Child Psychiatry
Philippe JEAMMET 149

Scientific Advances in Neonatology since the Year 2000
Hugo LAGERCRANTZ 163

Present and Future in Vaccinology
Stanley PLOTKIN 173

Clinical Approach to Inborn Metabolic Diseases: an Update
Jean-Marie SAUDUBRAY 181

Progress in Paediatric Endocrinology 2001-2006
Martin O. SAVAGE 197

Nutrition in Children: from Calories to Function
Yvan VANDENPLAS, *Silvia* SALVATORE,
Bruno HAUSER, *Jean de* SCHEPPER 207

Progrès récents en pédiatrie générale

Les progrès récents en gastroentérologie

Samy CADRANEL*

*Service de gastroentérologie, Hôpital Universitaire des Enfants Reine Fabiola,
Université Libre de Bruxelles, Bruxelles, Belgique*

La gastroentérologie pédiatrique n'est reconnue comme une spécialité que depuis une trentaine d'années. Au-delà de la pathologie gastroentérologique à proprement parler, comme la diarrhée et la malnutrition, les progrès réalisés dans ce domaine ont notamment mis en évidence l'importance du tube digestif en immunologie.

Le reflux gastro-œsophagien

Depuis que les ulcères gastroduodénaux ont quasiment disparu, le reflux gastro-œsophagien (RGO) représente au moins la moitié des motifs de consultation en gastroentérologie de l'adulte.
En pédiatrie, de par sa grande fréquence, le RGO reste également un problème.

* Rédaction : Catherine Faber, d'après la communication de Samy Cadranel au Colloque Charles Nicolle de Rouen.
Article publié préalablement dans *Médecine et Enfance*.

Considéré comme physiologique chez le nourrisson, il ne nécessite pas de traitement spécifique dans les cas non compliqués. Cependant, la mauvaise acceptation des régurgitations par les parents a conduit à la commercialisation de formules lactées antirégurgitation. Leur efficacité a été démontrée par une étude randomisée selon laquelle il est préférable d'utiliser une formule épaissie à 0,35 g/ml [1].

Les conséquences potentielles du RGO non traité sont évoquées de longue date. D'après une étude publiée à la fin des années cinquante, à l'âge de quatre ans, 10 % des enfants non traités présentent des complications et 30 % ont des symptômes persistants [2]. En ce qui concerne les symptômes extradigestifs du RGO, la revue des dossiers de 1980 patients âgés de deux à dix-huit ans et de 7 920 contrôles confirme l'existence d'une corrélation positive avec les infections respiratoires, sauf pour l'otite moyenne aiguë [3]. Il est possible de déterminer de manière plus objective la relation entre RGO et maladie respiratoire à l'aide du pH mesuré au niveau de la muqueuse nasale, qui apparaît comme un test ayant de bonnes sensibilité, spécificité et valeur prédictive positive [4].

Sur le plan thérapeutique, après une très large utilisation en première intention dans le RGO, les prokinétiques ont pratiquement disparu dans cette indication. Il n'est désormais possible de les utiliser que dans des conditions très précises, en milieu hospitalo-universitaire. Le Prépulsid® (cisapride) peut être prescrit selon certaines règles, mais certainement pas comme traitement antirégurgitation. Il était parfois associé au Gaviscon®, ce qui n'a aucun sens car ce dernier n'agit que lorsque le contenu de l'estomac est acide.

En l'absence de prokinétiques efficaces et facilement disponibles, les antiacides de type anti-H2 et inhibiteurs de la pompe à protons (IPP) sont apparus comme une alternative. D'après plusieurs études incluant des enfants, les IPP sont plus efficaces que les anti-H2 sur les symptômes de RGO et la cicatrisation des œsophagites érosives. Cependant, les auteurs d'une revue sur l'importance des IPP ont constaté que ces médicaments étaient prescrits de façon presque rituelle [5]. Cette large utilisation n'est pas opportune compte tenu de leurs effets secondaires, de la diversité et de la connaissance incomplète de leurs mécanismes d'action et, surtout, de leurs conséquences potentielles sur la microflore. Une étude italienne menée sur des enfants de moins de sept ans a montré que l'utilisation d'antisécrétoires et d'IPP s'accompagne d'un risque accru de gastroentérite aiguë et de pneumonie [6]. Cet effet semble persister même après arrêt du traitement. Des polypes gastriques hyperplasiques ont été décrits chez des adultes traités par IPP. Mais ils sont peu importants, réversibles et jamais néoplasiques.

Les GABA agonistes (baclofène) peuvent être utilisés chez les enfants présentant des troubles neurologiques qui sont sujets à des œsophagites gravissimes difficiles à traiter aussi bien médicalement que chirurgicalement [7]. Testé dans une petite série (n = 8), le baclofène a donné de bons résultats, avec une réduction de la fréquence des vomissements et du nombre total de reflux acides [8]. Ce traitement est certainement appelé à se développer dans le RGO.

Sur le plan physiopathologique, on dispose d'un nombre croissant de données sur l'effet délétère du reflux biliaire au niveau de la muqueuse œsophagienne. Les résultats de la surveillance du pH œsophagien et de la bilirubine chez 65 enfants ont mis en évidence une relation entre l'augmentation des reflux à la fois biliaires et acides et l'évolution vers une œsophagite sévère [9]. Enfin, une nouvelle technique combinant la pHmétrie et l'impédancemétrie pourrait dans l'avenir supplanter la pHmétrie œsophagienne ambulatoire des vingt-quatre heures [10]. Elle permet de caractériser la proportion des reflux acides et non acides chez les enfants avec suspicion de RGO et détecte un plus grand nombre de reflux que la pHmétrie. On attend de cette technique une amélioration de la connaissance des mécanismes physiopathologiques du RGO.

L'œsophagite à éosinophiles

Présentée comme une nouvelle entité, l'œsophagite à éosinophiles est, en fait, connue depuis le début des années 80. Elle se caractérise par une infiltration éosinophilique de l'épithélium ou des tissus profonds de l'œsophage, à raison de plus de 20 éosinophiles par champ. Sa symptomatologie est la même que celle du RGO, mais la pHmétrie est habituellement normale et elle répond peu aux traitements antireflux. Deux points importants doivent être connus : d'une part, la très large prédominance masculine [11] et, d'autre part, l'absence fréquente de RGO. La fréquence des antécédents allergiques ainsi que la bonne réponse aux traitements antiallergiques plaident en faveur d'une origine allergique de l'œsophagite à éosinophiles [12]. Son diagnostic doit être évoqué chez un enfant qui présente des symptômes persistants présumés dus à un RGO et ne répondant pas aux traitements antireflux. Une muqueuse normale à l'endoscopie ne doit pas dispenser de la réalisation de biopsies pour études histopathologiques [13]. Dans le traitement des œsophagites à éosinophiles, la première étape est d'éviter les allergies alimentaires. Malgré des effets bénéfiques bien documentés chez la plupart des patients avec symptômes intermittents, les corticoïdes oraux au long cours ne sont pas justifiés [14]. En revanche, cette œsophagite peut être améliorée par des corticoïdes locaux [15]. Les antileucotriènes, comme le montelukast, ont donné des résultats prometteurs dans cette indication.

Les œsophagites caustiques

Les accidents d'ingestion de produits caustiques acides ou alcalins posent des problèmes importants dans le monde, en particulier dans les pays défavorisés. Au Caire, ville qui compte 17 millions d'habitants, on recense une centaine de cas graves par mois.

Le Groupe francophone de gastroentérologie, hépatologie et nutrition pédiatriques a mis en place un protocole simple visant à prévenir les sténoses secondaires par l'administration de mégadoses de corticoïdes aussi tôt que possible après l'ingestion du produit caustique : méthylprednisolone 1 000 mg/1,73 m² en bolus en perfusion IV pendant trois heures pendant six jours [16]. Évaluée dans une étude multicentrique sur 43 petits patients et 17 contrôles, cette stratégie a donné de bons résultats (seulement 30 % de sténose), confirmant ainsi les données issues de travaux expérimentaux et les observations faites chez l'enfant il y a une dizaine d'années. Des résultats intéressants ont également été notés dans une étude tunisienne sur 26 enfants [17].

En ce qui concerne les dilatations endoscopiques, des techniques utilisant des stents ou des ballonnets ont été développées [18, 19]. L'objectif est de maintenir l'œsophage en position dilatée durant tout le processus de cicatrisation.
Enfin, l'application locale de mitomycine a été proposée récemment pour stabiliser ou réduire le nombre de dilatations nécessaires [20].

Helicobacter pylori

Si la transmission de l'infection à *Helicobacter pylori* est mal connue, on considère, sur la base de diverses études, que son acquisition a lieu dans l'enfance, en particulier dans les pays en développement [21]. Les résultats concordants d'études menées dans plusieurs pays aux conditions climatiques très différentes ont permis d'incriminer H pylori dans l'anémie sidéroblastique : en Turquie [22], en Alaska [23], en Colombie [24] et au Canada [25]. En revanche, le rôle de l'infection à H pylori sur la taille définitive, évoqué par plusieurs auteurs, est très difficile à prouver en raison de facteurs confondants liés à la promiscuité et aux mauvaises conditions socioéconomiques des populations dans lesquelles ce constat a été fait. Une autre donnée récente intéressante, surtout pour les pays défavorisés, est l'effet protecteur de l'allaitement maternel prolongé contre l'infection par cette bactérie [26].

Dans le traitement de première ligne de la gastrite à *H pylori*, les sels de bismuth (efficaces et peu coûteux) utilisés dans les années 80 et 90 ont été progressivement remplacés par l'association de deux antibiotiques et d'un IPP. La mauvaise réputation du bismuth vient de la description de cas d'encéphalopathie chez des enfants traités. Mais ces cas sont liés à la formulation et non à la molécule elle-même. En effet, les encéphalopathies ont été observées avec les nitrate et sous-galate de bismuth, jamais avec le sous-citrate de bismuth.

La trithérapie antibiotiques-IPP donne des taux d'éradication plus bas chez l'enfant que chez l'adulte [27]. Avec deux antibiotiques, le germe n'est éradiqué que dans 10 % des cas, mais ce taux atteint 80 % si un IPP est ajouté. Le coût élevé de la trithérapie, ainsi que l'augmentation des résistances des souches à la clarithromycine [28] constituent un obstacle à son utilisation large. La solution serait un vaccin, attendu depuis vingt ans.
D'autres pistes thérapeutiques sont explorées :
– les pré- et probiotiques : *Clostridium butyricum* n'a de valeur que par son effet de diminution des effets secondaires gastro-intestinaux [29] ; *Saccharomyces boulardii* participe à la réduction de la charge bactérienne [30] et permettrait donc, administré avant le traitement, d'utiliser moins d'antibiotiques ;
– des plantes culinaires et médicinales dotées de propriétés bactéricides (*in vitro*) et antiadhésives comme la réglisse [31], le cumin, le gingembre, l'origan, l'airelle…
Une autre donnée récente importante est la mise en évidence par des auteurs japonais d'une atrophie de la muqueuse gastrique au niveau de l'antre et du corps chez, respectivement, 10 % et 4 % des enfants infectés par *H pylori* et d'une métaplasie intestinale chez 4 % [32]. Ces données, apparemment constatées également en Afrique du Nord (données personnelles) battent en brèche l'idée selon laquelle la constitution d'une atrophie gastrique nécessite des années.

Les MICI

Le rôle des facteurs environnementaux dans l'apparition des maladies inflammatoires chroniques intestinales (MICI) apparaît de plus en plus important. L'hypothèse hygiénique est confortée par des données expérimentales montrant que les parasitoses (helminthes) entraînent des modifications de l'immunité du tube digestif [33]. Elles protègent contre l'inflammation gastro-intestinale médiée par les cellules T helper de type 1 comme la maladie de Crohn.

En ce qui concerne les nouveautés thérapeutiques, les anti-TNF alpha sont une grande découverte scientifique de ces cinq dernières années et le premier traitement ciblé sur un des mécanismes physiopathologiques des MICI. Ils ont été testés avec de bons résultats dans deux grandes séries pédiatriques, l'une américaine [34], l'autre européenne [35]. Les premiers résultats de l'hormone de croissance pour diminuer l'impact de la corticothérapie sont relativement prometteurs. Il faut toutefois garder à l'esprit leur implication dans des transformations malignes.

Les greffes d'hépatocytes

Plus de 1 000 transplantations hépatiques ont été réalisées chez des enfants dans un centre belge. Toutefois, de grands espoirs sont actuellement fondés sur la transplantation de cellules hépatiques plutôt que la greffe d'organe. Une banque d'hépatocytes est en projet. Elle permettra de fournir des cellules aux enfants arrivant avec une maladie métabolique décompensée notamment les anomalies du cycle de l'urée, la glycogénose type I, la maladie de Refsum, la maladie de Criggler-Najjar et la déficience en facteur VII. L'utilisation des hépatocytes peut être envisagée dans toutes les affections dans lesquelles le foie joue un rôle [36]. Dans la phénylcétonurie, par exemple, quelques cellules feraient passer le métabolisme de la phénylalanine de 0 à 5-10 %, soit un taux suffisant pour maintenir les enfants en bon état tout en ayant une alimentation normale.

Références

1. Miyazawa R, Tomomasa T, Kaneko H, Morikawa A. Effect of locust bean gum in anti-regurgitant milk on the regurgitation in uncomplicated gastrœsophageal reflux. *J Pediatr Gastroenterol Nutr* 2004 ; 38 : 479-83.
2. Carre I.J. The natural history of the partial thoracic stomach (hiatus hernia) in children. *Arch Dis Child* 1959 ; 34 : 344-53.
3. El-Serag HB, Gilger M, Kuebeler M, Rabeneck L. Extraesophageal associations of gastrœsophageal reflux disease in children without neurologic defects. *Gastroenterology* 2001 ; 121 : 1294-9.
4. Junqueria JC. Nasopharingeal pH as diagnostic test to confirm respiratory disease secondary to gastrœsophageal reflux. *J Pediatr Gastroenterol Nutr* 2005 ; 41 suppl. 1 : S79-80.
5. Scaillon M, Cadranel S. Safety data required for proton-pump inhibitor use in children. *J Pediatr Gastroenterol Nutr* 2002 ; 35 : 113-8.
6. Canani RB, Cirillo P, Roggero P, *et al.* Working Group on Intestinal Infections of the Italian Society of Pediatric Gastroenterology, Hepatology and Nutrition (SIGENP). Therapy with gastric acidity inhibitors increases the risk of acute gastroenteritis and community-acquired pneumonia in children. *Pediatrics* 2006 ; 117 : 817-20.
7. Lidums I, Lehmann A, Checklin H, *et al.* Control of transient lower esophageal sphincter relaxations and reflux by the GABA (B) agonist baclofen in normal subjects. *Gastroenterology* 2000 ; 118 : 7-13.

8. Kawai M, Kawahara H, Hirayama S, et al. Effect of baclofen on emesis and 24-hour œsophageal pH in neurologically impaired children with gastrœsophageal reflux disease. *J Pediatr* 2004 ; 38 : 317-23.
9. Orel R, Markovic S. Bile in the oesophagus : a factor in the pathogenesis of reflux esophagitis in children. *J Pediat Gastroenterol Nutr* 2003 ; 36 : 266-73.
10. Condino A, Sondheimer J, Pan Z, et al. Evaluation of infantile acid and non acid gastrœsophageal relfux using combined pH monitoring and impedance measurement. *J Pediatr Gastroenterol Nutr* 2006 ; 42 : 16-21.
11. Fox V, Nurko S, Furuta G. Eosinophilic esophagitis : it's not just kid's staff. *Gastrointest Endosc* 2002 ; 56 : 260-70.
12. Martin de Carpi J, Varea V, Gómez M, et al. Eosinophilic esophagitis : increasing prevalence or best recognized ? *J Pediatr Gastroenterol Nutr* 2004 ; 39 suppl. 1 : S240-1.
13. Cadranel S, Scaillon M, Segers V. Eosinophilic esophagitis, another reason for systematic endoscopic biopsies. *J Pediatr Gastroenterol Nutr* 2004 ; 39 Suppl 1 : S503-4.
14. Cheung KM, Oliver MR, Cameron DJS, et al. Esophageal eosinophilia in children with dysphagia. *J Pediatr Gastroenterol Nutr* 2003 ; 37 : 498-503.
15. Teitelbaum JE, Fox VL, Twarog FJ. et al. Eosinophilic esophagitis in children : immunopathological analysis and response to fluticasone proprionate. *J Pediatr Gastroenterol Nutr* 2002 ; 122 : 1216-25.
16. Breton A, Olives JP, Cadranel P, et al. Management of severe caustic esophageal burns in children with very high doses of steroids. *J Pediatr Gastroenterol Nutr* 2004 ; 39 suppl. 1 : S458.
17. Boukthir S, Fetni I, Mrad SM, et al. High doses of steroids in the management of caustic esophagaeal burns in children. *Arch Pediatr* 2004 ; 11 : 13-7.
18. Broto J, Asensio M, Vernet MG. Results of a new technique in the treatment of severe esophageal stenose in children : Poliflex stent. *J Pediatr Gastroenterol Nutr* 2003 ; 37 : 203-6.
19. Van Der Zee DC, Bax NM, De Schryver JE, Beek FJ. Indwelling balloon dilatation for esophageal stenosis in infants. *J Pediatr Gastroenterol Nutr* 2006 ; 42 : 437-9.
20. Uhlen S, Fayoux P, Vachin F, et al. Mitomycin C : an alternative conservative treatment for refractory esophageal stricture in children ? *Endoscopy* 2006 ; 38 : 404-7.
21. Rocha GA, Rocha AM, Silva LD, et al. Transmission of Helicobacter pylori infection in families of preschool-aged children from Minas Gerais, Brazil. *Trop Med Int Health* 2003 ; 8 : 987-91.
22. Baysoy G, Ertem D, Ademoglu E, et al. Gastric histopathology, iron status and iron deficiency anemia in children with Helicobacter pylori infection. *Pediatr Gastroenterol Nutr* 2004 ; 38 : 146-51.
23. Bagget HC, Parkinson AJ, Muth PT, et al. Endemic iron deficiency associated with Helicobacter pylori infection among school-aged children in Alaska. *Pediatrics* 2006 ; 117 : 396-404.
24. Mera RM, Correa P, Fontham EE, et al. Effects of a new Helicobacter pylori infection on height and weight in Colombian children. *Ann Epidemiol* 2006 ; 16 : 347-51.
25. Moayyedi P, Forman D, Duffett S, and HELP Study Group. Association between Helicobacter pylori infection and adult height. *Eur J Epidemiol* 2005 ; 20 : 455-65.
26. Pearce MS, Thomas JE, Campbell DI, Parker L. Does increased duration of exclusive breast-feeding protect against Helicobacter pylori Infection ? The Newcastle Thousand Families Cohort Study at age 49-51 years. *J Pediatr Gastroenterol Nutr* 2005 ; 41 : 617-20.
27. Gottrand F, Kalach N, Spyckerelle C, et al. Omeprazole combined with amoxicillin and clarithromycin in the eradication of Helicobacter pylori in children with gastritis : A prospective randomized double-blind trial. *J Pediatr* 2001 ; 139 : 664-8.
28. Koletzko S, Richy F, Bontems P, et al. Prospective multicentre study on antibiotic resistance of Helicobacter pylori strains obtained from children living in Europe. *Gut* 2006 ; 55 : 1711-6.
29. Shimbo I, Yamaguchi T, Odaka T, et al. Effect of Clostridium butyricum on fecal flora in Helicobacter pylori eradication therapy. *World J Gastroenterol*, 2005 ; 11 : 7520-4.
30. Gotteland M, Poliak L, Cruchet S, Brunser O. Effect of regular ingestion of Saccharomyces boulardii plus inulin or Lactobacillus acidophilus LB in children colonized by Helicobacter pylori. *Acta Paediatr* 2005 ; 94 : 1747-51.

31. O'Mahonny R, Al-Khtheeri H, Weerasekera D, *et al.* Bactericidal and anti-adhesive properties of culinary and medicinal plants against Helicobacter pylori. *World J Gastroenterol*, 2005 ; 11 : 7499-507.
32. Kato S, Nakajima S, Nishino Y, *et al.* Association between gastric atrophy and Helicobacter pylori infection in Japanese children : a retrospective multicenter study. *Dig Dis Sci*, 2006 ; 51 : 99-104.
33. Amre DK, Lambrette P, Law L, *et al.* Investigating the hygiene hypothesis as a risk factor in pediatric onset Crohn's disease : a case-control study. *Am J Gastroenterol* 2006 ; 101 : 1005-11.
34. Friesen CA, Calabro C, Christenson K, *et al.* Safety of infliximab treatment in pediatric patients with inflammatory bowel disease. *J Pediatr Gastroenterol Nutr* 2004 ; 39 : 265-9.
35. Lamireau T, Cezard JP, Dabadie A, *et al.* Efficacy and tolerance of infliximab in children and adolescents with Crohn's disease. *Inflamm Bowel Dis* 2004 ; 10 : 745-50.
36. Nussler A, Konig S, Ott M, *et al.* Present status and perspectives of cell-based therapies for liver diseases. *J Hepatol* 2006 ; 45 : 144-59.

Les progrès récents en épileptologie

*Olivier DULAC**

Service de Neuropédiatrie, Hôpital Necker-Enfants Malades, Paris, France

Depuis 2000, les épilepsies ont fait l'objet de très nombreuses publications, comme le confirme la recherche de données bibliographiques sur PubMed avec les mots « epilepsy » et « children ». Au cours des cinq dernières années, le nombre de références indexées dans cette base atteint 5 000. Les progrès accomplis pouvant donc difficilement être évoqués de façon exhaustive, cet article porte sur les nouvelles données acquises dans certains domaines de l'épileptologie pédiatrique.

Découvertes génétiques

Le syndrome de Dravet

En 2001, une équipe belge a identifié le gène associé au syndrome de Dravet [1]. Ce syndrome est une forme rare, mais extrêmement grave, de convulsions fébriles. Il débute au milieu de la première année de vie et évolue vers une épilepsie myoclo-

---

* Rédaction : Catherine Faber, d'après la communication d'Olivier Dulac au Colloque Charles Nicolle de Rouen.

nique. Des mutations du gène *SCN1A* ont été identifiées grâce à des travaux menés sur une grande famille française dont des membres présentaient un tableau associant des convulsions fébriles, une épilepsie généralisée idiopathique et des « convulsions fébriles plus » (persistant après l'âge de six ans). Les auteurs ont rapporté les sept premiers cas qui, tous, étaient porteurs de mutations du gène *SCN1A* qui code pour un canal sodium.

Cette découverte n'a pas d'implication sur le plan du diagnostic, car si les mutations sont présentes chez 100 % des patients de la série belge, des études ultérieures ont révélé des proportions inférieures, de 60 à 80 %, et même de 35 % dans des travaux de Généthon III [2]. Ces différences expliquent le risque d'erreurs par défaut, mais aussi par excès. Le même type de mutation a, en effet, été retrouvé dans une autre forme d'épilepsie caractérisée par une épilepsie généralisée sévère du nourrisson sans myoclonies [3].

Sur le plan thérapeutique également, les implications sont discutables. L'histoire des enfants atteints montre qu'ils développent un état de mal dans les six mois. Pour définir la stratégie thérapeutique, les mutations devraient donc être recherchées dans ce délai ; ce qui n'est pas le cas. Cette découverte illustre les perversions de certaines avancées de la génétique. Dans la pratique, les indications des traitements doivent reposer sur la clinique et non sur la génétique. Le même problème se pose pour le conseil génétique. Certaines familles ont deux enfants atteints mais avec des parents sans la mutation ou avec une chimère. De plus, il y a un nombre très élevé de mutations et pas de point chaud de mutation. Leur mise en évidence représente donc un travail considérable. Enfin, les mutations du gène *SCN1A* ne sont pas prédictives du syndrome de Dravet.

La découverte de ces mutations a tout de même un intérêt en termes de reconnaissance du syndrome de Dravet et d'explication de la maladie aux parents. Elle a aussi permis, d'une part, de confirmer la distinction entre certaines formes d'épilepsie qui avaient toutes été regroupées et l'épilepsie myoclono-astatique, et, d'autre part, d'exclure la responsabilité de vaccins (encéphalopathie vaccinale).

Les autres pathologies monogéniques

Des anomalies génétiques ont été découvertes dans d'autres maladies monogéniques :
– des mutations du gène *SCN2A* dans les convulsions néonatales familiales bénignes qui apparaissent entre l'âge de deux et sept mois [4] et dans des formes de convulsions infantiles bénignes [5] ;
– des mutations *de novo* du gène *ARX* dans une forme d'épilepsie avec crises myocloniques ou spasmes infantiles [6] ;

– des mutations *de novo* du gène CDKL5 dans une épilepsie caractérisée par des spasmes précédés de crises toniques, avant l'âge de trois mois [7].

Maladies métaboliques et épilepsie

Une absence congénitale d'un transporteur mitochondrial du glutamate a été rapportée récemment dans deux familles [8]. Cette maladie à transmission autosomique récessive se manifeste par une encéphalopathie myoclonique néonatale. À l'instar de l'encéphalopathie glycinique et des épilepsies pyridoxino-dépendante et pyridoxal phosphate-dépendante, elle se caractérise par une augmentation du ratio glutamate/GABA. Chez l'animal, le blocage expérimental des transporteurs du glutamate aboutit au même tableau. On sait qu'un métabolisme du glutamate normal est capital pour plusieurs fonctions dont celle du système nerveux central. L'identification de cette cause d'épilepsie myoclonique précoce souligne l'importance du métabolisme mitochondrial et ouvre une nouvelle voie de recherche physiopathologique dans les épilepsies sévères néonatales.

Dans le syndrome d'Alpers, des travaux publiés en 2005 ont permis d'impliquer des mutations du gène *pol-gamma* [9]. Aucun des six patients décrits (qui appartenaient à des familles différentes) ne présentaient d'anomalies de la chaîne respiratoire. Ces mutations sont responsables de l'importante déplétion de l'ADN mitochondrial qui caractérise le syndrome. Il a également été montré, récemment, que des spasmes infantiles, avec à l'IRM un hypersignal du ganglion basal, peuvent révéler une mitochondriopathie due à la mutation de l'ADN mitochondrial T8993G (celle du syndrome NARP : neuropathie, ataxie, rétinite pigmentaire) [10]. Bien qu'étant une maladie mitochondriale, elle doit être traitée comme des spasmes infantiles : ceux-ci sont sensibles aux corticoïdes et au vigabatrin.

Maturation cérébrale et épilepsie

Il existe indiscutablement une relation entre maturation cérébrale et épilepsie. L'épilepsie retarde la maturation cérébrale, et plus le cerveau est immature, plus le risque de pharmacorésistance est élevé. L'étude d'EEG pédiatriques a montré que les foyers de pointes-ondes prédominent plus souvent au niveau de l'hémisphère gauche avant l'âge de cinq ans et droit au-delà de cet âge [11], ce qui conforte des données selon lesquelles la maturation de l'hémisphère gauche est plus tardive.

Plusieurs arguments indiquent que la maturation cérébrale contribue largement à l'épileptogenèse. Au cours de la période précoce de la vie, le GABA est un excitateur ; le seul neurotransmetteur excitateur puisque le NMDA est sous contrôle strict via les transporteurs du glutamate. L'augmentation de la transmission NMDA entraîne une épilepsie néonatale avec myoclonies et « *suppression-bursts* » (alternance de bouffées de pointes de grande amplitude et d'EEG plat). En période néonatale, les aspects EEG de ce type sont dus à un manque d'inhibition GABA. Les anomalies de la neurotransmission synaptique impliquent différentes aires, notamment l'aire motrice à terme (activité myoclonique), les aires pariéto-occipitales durant la petite enfance (agénésie visuelle dans le syndrome de West) et les lobes frontaux durant l'enfance (syndrome de Lennox-Gastaut). On sait aussi que la myéline est nécessaire pour la synchronisation interhémisphérique et que la myélinisation incomplète avant l'âge de dix-huit mois est responsable de l'asynchronie des pointes dans l'hypsarythmie. Concernant l'apparition progressive des connexions à distance entre la moelle épinière et le moteur, et entre le néocortex et l'hippocampe, divers points peuvent être soulignés, parmi lesquels les conséquences potentielles du développement prématuré des voies hippocampo-néocorticales. Ce phénomène pourrait provoquer la production par l'hippocampe d'un écho sur un cortex hyperexcitable et, de ce fait, être à l'origine d'une encéphalopathie épileptique sévère de description récente [12]. La maladie apparaît chez un enfant d'âge scolaire ayant un développement normal. Elle débute par un état de mal épileptique prolongé, souvent déclenché par une fièvre, et évolue vers une épilepsie intraitable accompagnée d'une détérioration cognitive sévère.

Les traitements médicamenteux

Ces cinq dernières années ont vu la confirmation de l'efficacité du vigabatrin dans les spasmes infantiles [13]. Chez l'enfant, ce médicament a une toxicité rétinienne qui est moindre que chez l'adulte [14].

Les observations de la pratique quotidienne ont fait apparaître l'utilité du topiramate (médicament bien étudié chez l'adulte) dans les spasmes infantiles et le syndrome de Dravet. Enfin, la mise à disposition des médecins d'une forme de microgranules à absorption différée de valproate de sodium (Micropakine®) représente un progrès majeur en épileptologie pédiatrique.

Références

1. Claes L, Del-Favero J, Ceulemans B, et al. De novo mutations in the sodium-channel gene SCN1A cause severe myoclonic epilepsy of infancy. *Am J Hum Genet* 2001 ; 68 : 1327-32.
2. Nabbout R, Gennaro E, Dalla Bernardina B, et al. Spectrum of SCN1A mutations in severe myoclonic epilepsy of infancy. *Neurology* 2003 ; 60 : 1961-7.
3. Fujiwara T, Sugawara T, Mazaki-Miyazaki E, et al. Mutations of sodium channel alpha subunit type 1 (SCN1A) in intractable childhood epilepsies with frequent generalized tonic-clonic seizures. *Brain* 2003 ; 126 : 531-46.
4. Heron SE, Crossland KM, Andermann E, et al. Sodium-channel defects in benign familial neonatal-infantile seizures. *Lancet* 2002 ; 360 : 851-2.
5. Striano P, Bordo L, Lispi ML, et al. A novel SCN2A mutation in family with benign familial infantile seizures. *Epilepsia* 2006 ; 47 : 218-20.
6. Scheffer IE, Wallace RH, Phillips FL, et al. X-linked myoclonic epilepsy with spasticity and intellectual disability : mutation in the homeobox gene ARX. *Neurology* 2002 ; 59 : 348-56.
7. Evans JC, Archer HL, Colley JP, et al. Early onset seizures and Rett-like features associated with mutations in CDKL5. *Eur J Hum Genet* 2005 ; 13 : 1113-20.
8. Molinari F, Raas-Rothschild A, Rio M, et al. Impaired mitochondrial glutamate transport in utosomal recessive neonatal myoclonic epilepsy. *Am J Hum Genet* 2005 ; 76 : 334-9.
9. Nguyen KV, Ostergaard E, Ravn SH, et al. POLG mutations in Alpers syndrome. *Neurology* 2005 ; 65 : 1493-95.
10. Desguerre I, Pinton F, Nabbout R, et al. Infantile spasms with basal ganglia MRI hypersignal may reveal mitochondrial disorder due to T8993G MT DNA mutation. *Neuropediatrics* 2003 ; 34 : 265-69.
11. Doherty MJ, Simon E, De Menezes MS, et al. When might hemispheric favouring of epileptiform discharges begin ? *Seizure* 2003 ; 12 : 595-8.
12. Mikaeloff Y, Jambaque I, Hertz-Pannier L, et al. Devastating epileptic encephalopathy in school-aged children (DESC) : A pseudo encephalitis. *Epilepsy Res* 2006 ; 69 : 67-79.
13. Elterman RD, Shields WD, Mansfield KA, Nakagawa J. Randomized trial of vigabatrin in patients with infantile spasms. *Neurology* 2001 ; 57 : 1416-21.
14. Vanhatalo S, Nousiainen I, Eriksson K, et al. Visual field constriction in 91 Finnish children treated with vigabatrin. *Epilepsia* 2002 ; 43 : 748-56.
15. Eisermann MM, DeLaRaillere A, Dellatolas G, et al. Infantile spasms in Down syndrome-effects of delayed anticonvulsive treatment. Epilepsy Res 2003 ; 55 : 21-7.

Les progrès récents dans le métabolisme osseux et phosphocalcique chez l'enfant

*Michèle GARABÉDIAN**

Inserm U561, Hôpital Saint-Vincent-de-Paul, Paris, France

De nombreuses études sur les métabolismes osseux et phosphocalcique ont été publiées depuis 2000. Les principaux points marquants de ces dernières années sont la remise en question d'un dogme concernant les effets du calcium et des produits laitiers sur l'os, la mise en évidence d'un nouveau système de communication entre les ostéoblastes et les ostéoclastes, l'identification de toute une série de gènes responsables de maladies osseuses chez l'enfant (et chez l'adulte) et la découverte d'une troisième hormone impliquée dans le métabolisme du phosphate.

Les effets du calcium et des produits laitiers sur l'os

Jusqu'en 2000, le rôle du calcium et/ou des produits laitiers pour la santé osseuse pendant l'enfance et l'adolescence, puis pour la vie ultérieure semblaient clairs. À

* Rédaction : Catherine Faber, d'après la communication de Michèle Garabédian au Colloque Charles Nicolle de Rouen.

partir de cette date, plusieurs publications sont venues remettre en cause le dogme sur lequel reposent les apports recommandés en calcium. L'une, qui a repris cent trente-neuf études sorties depuis 1975, est en faveur de cette certitude [1]. Mais deux autres revues ont donné des résultats contradictoires. La première, publiée la même année, a analysé cinquante-sept études et conclut que les preuves sont insuffisantes pour soutenir les recommandations d'apports quotidiens de produits laitiers pour avoir une bonne santé osseuse [2]. La seconde, qui date de 2005 et a porté sur cinquante-huit études, indique qu'il y a peu de preuves justifiant les recommandations actuelles d'une augmentation des apports de produits laitiers pour accroître la masse osseuse et la minéralisation chez l'enfant et l'adolescent [3].

À la lueur des données disponibles, on s'aperçoit donc que, en 2006, il n'y a pas de démonstration formelle de la pertinence des apports recommandés ou même des besoins nutritionnels en calcium pour une bonne minéralisation pendant l'enfance et l'adolescence. En revanche, il apparaît clairement qu'une carence en calcium ou une faible consommation de produits laitiers durant cette période de la vie diminue le gain de masse osseuse. Elle affecte non seulement la minéralisation du squelette mais aussi la taille et la forme des os (diamètre, épaisseur…) et, de ce fait, a un impact négatif sur la taille et le risque fracturaire à l'âge adulte.

Lait pendant la croissance et ostéoporose/risque de fracture après la ménopause

Un autre point toujours à l'étude est le lien entre la consommation de calcium et de produits laitiers pendant l'enfance et l'adolescence, et l'ostéoporose postménopausique. Une relation entre cette consommation et le risque de fracture ou de tassements vertébraux après la ménopause avait été mise en évidence par un certain nombre d'études. Cependant, aucune d'entre elles n'avait pris en compte les apports calciques respectifs aux différentes étapes de la vie. Les résultats d'une étude utilisant les données de l'enquête NANHES III (*National Health and Nutrition Examination Survey*) menée sur des infirmières américaines permettent une approche plus précise de cette question [4]. Ses auteurs ont analysé la masse osseuse, la DMO, la taille des os et les fractures chez 3 251 femmes de vingt ans ou plus interrogées sur leurs apports calciques.
Ils ont observé que la consommation de lait pendant l'adolescence (13-17 ans) augmente de 2 à 3 % la densité minérale de la hanche chez la femme adulte jeune et après la ménopause. Mais cette consommation n'a aucun impact sur le risque fracturaire ni avant, ni après 50 ans. En revanche, une faible consommation de lait inférieure à 1 verre par semaine pendant l'enfance (5-12 ans) est associée à un risque de fracture non ostéoporotique deux fois plus élevé, avec un risque relatif de 2,02

(IC 95 % ; 1,13-3,59) chez les femmes de 0 à 49 ans et de 2,25 (IC 95 % ; 1,26-4) à partir de 50 ans.
Cette étude suggère donc que la consommation de lait pendant l'enfance et l'adolescence n'a pas un effet majeur sur la masse osseuse et la DMO des femmes adultes, qu'elles soient ménopausées ou non. En revanche, la prise de lait pendant l'enfance semble avoir un impact sur la taille et la forme des os, et donc sur le risque de fractures chez les femmes adultes.

La communication intercellulaire

Une découverte importante a été faite ces dernières années, celle d'un nouveau système de communication entre la lignée des ostéoblastes et des ostéoclastes. Il implique le récepteur RANK (*Receptor Activator of NF-Kappa B Ligand*) exprimé par les précurseurs des ostéclastes, ainsi que la cytokine RANK-L et l'ostéoprotégérine, produites par les ostéoblastes et les cellules stromales de la moelle osseuse [5]. RANK-L est un activateur majeur de la différenciation des précurseurs des ostéoclastes en ostéoclastes matures. Le système RANK/RANK-L a donc une activité pro-ostéoclastique. L'ostéoprotégérine (OPG) est un récepteur soluble produit par les ostéoblastes qui se lie avec RANK-L, l'empêchant d'être disponible pour son récepteur RANK. Cette protéine est un inhibiteur physiologique de la résorption osseuse. L'estradiol bloque la production de RANK-L et stimule celle de l'OPG. Les corticoïdes ont un effet exactement inverse.

Des avancées en génétique

Les recherches récentes ont permis d'identifier plusieurs gènes responsables de maladies osseuses et d'améliorer les connaissances de l'étiopathogénie de certaines d'entre elles.

Métabolisme osseux

Sont maintenant identifiés les gènes codant pour RANK (*TNF RSF 11A*) et pour l'OPG (*TNF RSF 11B*). Des mutations sur ces gènes altèrent les mécanismes de régulation du couplage ostéoblastes/ostéoclastes et sont responsables d'un remodelage osseux accéléré dans le cadre des maladies telles que la maladie de Paget de l'enfant et des formes familiales ou idiopathiques d'hyperphosphatasie. De nombreuses études en population pédiatrique sont en cours à la recherche d'un lien éventuel avec la maladie de Paget de l'adulte et sur l'association avec le risque d'ostéoporose.

D'autres gènes pour lesquels les connaissances ont progressé concernent la fonction de l'ostéoblaste :
CBFA-1/RUNX 2 code pour un facteur de différentiation et de maturation des ostéoblastes et des cellules du cartilage. On a découvert récemment des associations d'anomalies de *RUNX 2* avec une maladie, la dysplasie cléidocrânienne, des anomalies dentaires (malformations ou dents surnuméraires) et certaines ostéoporoses. De même, une association a été observée entre polymorphisme du gène *RUNX 2*, d'une part, et densité minimale osseuse et risques de fractures du poignet chez la femme âgée, d'autre part.

Des mutations de *TGF β1* (gène codant pour le *transforming growth factor beta 1*) ont été mises en évidence dans le syndrome de Camurati-Engelmann caractérisé par une hyperostase avec displasie diaphysaire. Comme *CBFA-1/RUNX 2*, il s'agit d'un gène connu depuis longtemps, mais qui a maintenant une traduction clinique.

Contrairement aux deux précédents, le gène *LRP 5* (gène codant pour la *low-density lipoprotein receptor related protein 5*) a été identifié récemment. On ne soupçonnait pas son lien avec l'os. Des analyses génétiques sur de grandes familles affectées par un syndrome associant une ostéoporose sévère et des pseudogliomes ont permis de découvrir l'association de cette maladie avec un locus dans le génome qui correspond à *LRP 5*. Outre le syndrome ostéoporose-pseudogliome, maladie très rare débutant dans l'enfance, des mutations perte-de-fonction de *LRP5* ont été retrouvées dans des formes d'ostéoporose juvénile, mais aussi dans des syndromes de forte masse osseuse, sans pseudogliomes. Pour ce gène, les progrès sont partis de la clinique pour aboutir à la conception d'un mécanisme insoupçonné d'activation de l'ostéoblaste, ouvrant la voie à une nouvelle approche thérapeutique de l'ostéoporose.

Des données récentes sur les ostéoclastes sont également disponibles. Les résultats observés sur des modèles de souris laissaient penser que, dans la plupart des ostéopétroses, ces cellules sont absentes. En fait, des travaux chez l'homme ont montré la présence d'ostéoclastes, mais non fonctionnels. Deux gènes identifiés depuis 2000 sont responsables de la plupart des ostéopétroses : *TCIRG1* et *CLCN7* qui codent, respectivement, pour une pompe à protons et pour un canal chlore. Le diagnostic des ostéopétroses est évident, ces données n'ont pas un intérêt majeur sur le plan du diagnostic génétique. Elles n'ouvrent pas non plus de champ de recherche très important.

Les avancées dans le domaine des protéines de la matrice concernent les dysplasies épiphysaires multiples dans lesquelles au moins cinq gènes ont été impliqués. Un autre gène en cause dans ce groupe de maladies a été identifié récemment : *MATN3* (matrilin-3). De façon plus anecdotique, la cause du chérubinisme est désormais connue : cette dysplasie fibro-osseuse bénigne de l'enfance peut être due à des mutations du gène *SH3BP2*.

Métabolisme calcique

Dans ce domaine, les progrès ont été plus modestes, tant sur le plan diagnostique que thérapeutique. Cependant plusieurs découvertes peuvent être signalées concernant les hyperparathyroïdies et hypoparathyroïdies.

Si un nouveau gène, *HRPT2*, a été ajouté en 2002 à la liste des gènes responsables d'hyperparathyroïdie, celui-ci n'est impliqué que dans les cas exceptionnels associant hyperparathyroïdie et tumeurs de la mâchoire. Dans la plupart des hyperparathyroïdies familiales, on trouve des anomalies, soit du gène *MEN 1* ou *MEN 2*, soit du gène *CaSR* codant pour le récepteur sensible au calcium – situé sur le chromosome 3 –, qui peut être le siège de mutations activatrices ou inhibitrices entraînant des hypo- ou des hypercalcémies, respectivement. Mais il apparaît maintenant que les hypercalcémies bénignes avec hypocalciurie ne sont pas toutes liées à des mutations du gène *CaSR*. Certaines le sont à des locus localisés sur le chromosome 19. À l'inverse, des anomalies du gène du récepteur du calcium ont été retrouvées dans une forme de syndrome de Bartter comportant, en plus des signes classiques du syndrome, une hypocalcémie et une hypercalciurie. Ainsi, le récepteur du calcium pourrait jouer un rôle dans la réabsorption du potassium.

En ce qui concerne les hypoparathyroïdies, le syndrome de DiGeorge et le syndrome vélo-cardio-facial, décrits depuis longtemps, sont associés à une microdélétion du chromosome 22 (22q11). Mais la ou les anomalies génétiques à l'origine de ces syndromes commencent seulement à être entrevues avec la mise en évidence du rôle capital joué par le gène *TBX1* dans cette région.

Enfin, en ce qui concerne la résistance à l'hormone parathyroïdienne (PTH, pseudo-hypoparathyroïdie), on sait depuis 2000, que le gène responsable, *GNAS1* (gène codant pour la protéine Gs alpha, intermédiaire obligatoire pour l'action des hormones ayant des récepteurs membranaires activant la voie de signalisation intracellulaire AMP cyclique dépendante), s'exprime différemment selon qu'il est d'origine maternelle ou paternelle. Lorsque le parent transmetteur est la mère, la pathologie est complète. S'il s'agit du père, l'hypocalcémie et la résistance à l'hormone parathyroïdienne sont absentes, car seul l'allèle maternel est exprimé au niveau du tubule proximal du rein, lieu d'action de cette hormone. Ce constat a permis de décrire une autre maladie associée à une mutation de GNAS1 avec défaut de l'allèle paternel : l'hétéroplasie osseuse progressive (HOP). Cette affection rare débute pendant l'enfance et se caractérise par des ossifications sous-cutanées évoluant progressivement. Elle peut être invalidante et, même, avoir une issue fatale par immobilisation totale du patient. L'HOP est causée par une différenciation excessive des cellules mésenchymateuse en ostéoblastes et se distingue donc de la myosite ossifiante.

La pseudohypoparathyroïdie de type 1b (PHP 1b) a également bénéficié des recherches de ces dernières années. On pensait qu'elle résultait d'une anomalie du gène du récepteur PTH/ PTHrP. Mais les tableaux cliniques résultant de ces anomalies concernent plutôt des anomalies de développement fœtal, chondrodysplasie de Blomstrand en cas de mutation perte-de-fonction, ou à l'inverse, des anomalies osseuses et calciques congénitales liées à une hypersensibilité à la PTH et au PTHrP (chondrodysplasie métaphysaire de Jansen), en cas de mutations gain-de-fonction. En fait, la cause actuellement la plus fréquente de PHPIb est un défaut d'expression de l'allèle maternel de GNAS1 au niveau rénal, en raison d'anomalies en amont de ce gène sur le chromosome 20q13.3 (défaut de méthylation ou délétion du gène STX16).

Métabolisme du phosphate : une troisième hormone

Décrit depuis une soixantaine d'années, le rachitisme hypophosphatémique familial – rachitisme vitamine D-résistant – se caractérise par un défaut de réabsorption proximale du phosphate associé à une mutation du gène PHEX.

Ces dernières années ont été marquées par de nouveaux développements concernant cette maladie, avec la découverte d'un troisième facteur (en plus de la PTH et de la vitamine D active) impliqué dans l'homéostasie du phosphate : la phosphatonine, et en particulier FGF23 [6]. Ce facteur synthétisé notamment par les ostéoblastes, inhibe, dans le tubule rénal proximal, la conversion de vitamine D en calcitriol et la résorption des phosphates en diminuant l'expression des cotransporteurs Npt2a et Npt2c. Il circule dans le sang sous une forme inactivée, clivée par des peptidases, notamment l'endopeptidase membranaire PHEX. On sait aujourd'hui que le rachitisme hypophosphatémique, dans ses formes à transmission dominante, est une maladie de l'ostéoblaste et non une maladie rénale.

Le rachitisme hypophosphatémique lié à l'X est dû à une mutation inactivatrice du gène *PHEX* entraînant une augmentation des taux de phosphatonine responsable de l'hypophosphatémie. Une autre forme de rachitisme hypophosphatémique, à transmission autosomique dominante, est liée à des anomalies du gène codant pour la phosphatonine FGF23 (*fibroblast growth factor 23*).

Enfin, une forme de rachitisme hypophosphatémique avec hypercalciurie a été identifiée chez des Bédouins en Israël et dans des familles turques en France. Une inactivation du gène *SLC34A3*, codant pour un cotransporteur sodium-phosphate Npt2c exprimé dans les cellules tubulaires rénales, vient d'être incriminée dans cette maladie autosomique récessive.

Les développements thérapeutiques

Sur le plan thérapeutique, deux évolutions sont à noter : d'une part, les résultats prometteurs des bisphosphonates pour le traitement des ostéoporoses liées à une résorption osseuse excessive chez l'enfant et, d'autre part, l'extension des indications de l'hormone de croissance aux enfants de petite taille souffrant de maladies de l'os ou du cartilage. Par ailleurs, l'introduction de « calcimimétiques » activant les récepteurs sensibles au calcium offre de nouvelles possibilités thérapeutiques pour le traitement des hyperparathyroïdies de l'enfant.

Références

1. Heaney RP. Calcium, dairy products and osteoporosis. *J Am Coll Nutr* 2000 ; 19 : 83S-99S.
2. Weinsier RL, Krumdieck CL. Dairy foods and bone health : examination of the evidence. *Am J Clin Nutr* 2000 ; 72 : 681-9.
3. Lanou AJ, Berkow SE, Barnard ND. Calcium, dairy products, and bone health in children and young adults : a reevaluation of the evidence. *Pediatrics* 2005 ; 115 : 736-43.
4. Kalkwarf HJ, Khoury JC, Lanphear BP. Milk intake during childhood and adolescence, adult bone density, and osteoporotic fractures in US women. *Am J Clin Nutr* 2003 ; 77 : 257-65.
5. Tanaka S. Signaling axis in osteoclast biology and therapeutic targeting in the RANK L/RANK/OPG system. *Am J Nephrol* 2007 ; 27 : 466-78. Erratum in: *Am J Nephrol* 2007 ; 27 : 54.
6. White KE, Larsson TM, Econs JM. The roles of specific genes implicated as circulating factors involved in normal and disordered phosphate homeostasis : Frizzled related-protein-4, matrix extracellular phosphoglycoprotein and fibroblast growth factor 23. *Endocr Rev* 2006 ; 27 : 221-41.

Développements récents en néphrologie pédiatrique

Jean-Pierre GUIGNARD

Unité de néphrologie, Service de pédiatrie, CHU Vaudois, Lausanne, Suisse

L'amélioration des soins cliniques apportés aux nouveau-nés, aux nourrissons et aux enfants est étroitement associée aux progrès réalisés grâce à l'expérimentation animale, aux études cliniques et à la mise sur le marché d'agents pharmacologiques efficaces. Ce chapitre a pour but de présenter quelques avancées récentes dans le domaine des affections rénales de l'enfant. Les progrès survenus en néphrologie pédiatrique sont souvent étroitement liés aux progrès réalisés chez l'adulte, tant du point de vue clinique que du point de vue expérimental.

Génétique

Des progrès récents ont été réalisés dans le domaine de la génétique des maladies rénales. De nombreux gènes ont été identifiés, et les conséquences de leur mutation clairement définies. C'est spécialement le cas pour certaines formes de syndrome néphrotique congénital [1], pour la néphronophtise ou l'hyperoxalurie primaire [2].

Évaluation du débit de filtration glomérulaire (DFG)

La filtration glomérulaire est généralement estimée sur la base de la créatinine plasmatique, ou mesurée par la clearance de la créatinine. Un nouveau marqueur du DFG, la cystatine C, a été mis sur le marché. Ce marqueur a été considéré par certains comme meilleur que la créatinine, notamment parce que sa concentration plasmatique paraissait indépendante de la masse musculaire et du sexe [3]. La cystatine est librement filtrée puis complètement réabsorbée par les tubules rénaux. Se retrouvant donc en quantité négligeable dans l'urine, elle n'est pas un marqueur classique du DFG, notamment parce que sa clearance urinaire ne peut évidemment pas être mesurée.

De nombreuses études ont tenté de valider la cystatine C comme marqueur du DFG. Très rares sont cependant celles qui ont utilisé le standard de référence pour cette validation, à savoir la clearance urinaire de l'inuline. Une grande étude portant sur 8 058 adultes a clairement démontré que le sexe masculin, un âge avancé, une surcharge pondérale, une mesure sérique élevée de la protéine C réactive ainsi que le tabagisme, étaient indépendamment associés à des concentrations sériques plus élevées de cystatine C, même après ajustement à la clearance de la créatinine [4]. La cystatine C paraît également être un mauvais marqueur du DFG chez les transplantés rénaux et/ou chez des patients sous corticothérapie [5]. Une étude récente chez l'enfant, utilisant la clearance urinaire de l'inuline comme mesure de référence du DFG, a démontré que la mesure de la concentration de la cystatine C était moins fiable que la formule de Schwartz pour estimer le DFG [6]. Le rapport coût/bénéfice de la cystatine C s'avère très élevé, la mesure de la cystatine C étant 12 fois plus onéreuse que celle de la créatinine. Contrairement à certaines affirmations, la cystatine C ne semble donc pas être un meilleur marqueur du DFG que la créatinine endogène. La généralisation de son utilisation ne peut donc être recommandée.

Prise en charge des maladies rénales

Syndrome néphrotique (SN)

L'utilisation d'un nouvel agent prometteur, le mycophenolate mofetil (MMF), permettra peut-être un meilleur contrôle du syndrome néphrotique, tout en diminuant les effets secondaires des traitements utilisés jusqu'ici. Le MMF est un inhibiteur sélectif et réversible de l'inosine-monophosphate-déhydrogénase ; il inhibe la synthèse « *de novo* » de purines. Il semble représenter une thérapie additionnelle intéressante en cas de SN. Chez les enfants présentant un SN corticodépendant ou corticorésistant et traités par prednisone, levamisole et/ou cyclophosphamide, l'administration de MMF a permis de diminuer significativement les doses de stéroïdes, avec amélioration consécutive de la croissance, de l'apparence physique ainsi que de la tension artérielle. Les effets bénéfiques du MMF ont été confirmés récemment dans une étude prospective chez des enfants présentant un SN corticodépendant [7]. La dose cible journalière utilisée était de 2 x 600 mg/m^2. Les effets secondaires associés à ce traitement ont été modérés, le plus souvent sous forme d'une gêne gastro-intestinale transitoire. L'efficacité évidente du MMF ainsi que son profil pharmacologique en font un agent de premier choix lors de syndromes néphrotiques corticodépendants nécessitant des doses élevées de stéroïdes. Des études soigneusement contrôlées permettront d'établir des protocoles d'utilisation optimale du MMF dans diverses formes de SN.

Insuffisance rénale chronique

Anémie

Le développement d'une érythropoïétine à longue durée d'action, darbepoïétine-alpha, dont la demi-vie moyenne est de 43 heures a amélioré la prise en charge des enfants anémiques. L'injection sous-cutanée de la darbepoïétine-alpha semble malheureusement plus douloureuse que celle de la traditionnelle érythropoïétine-bêta [8]. La mise prochaine sur le marché du Mircera®, activateur continu des récepteurs de l'érythropoïétine (*Continuous Erythropoietin Recepteur Activator* - CERA), permettra sans doute d'étendre encore davantage les espaces d'administration de l'érythropoïétine et de faciliter la prise en charge de l'anémie.

Ostéodystrophie rénale

Chélateurs du phosphate

L'hyperphosphatémie est un facteur-clé dans la pathogenèse de l'ostéodystrophie rénale. L'administration de chélateurs du phosphate est nécessaire chez la plupart des enfants dialysés. Les chélateurs à base d'aluminium font courir les risques de toxicité bien connus de l'aluminium tels qu'encéphalopathie, ostéomalacie, myopathie et anémie microcytaire. Les chélateurs à base de calcium augmentent le calcium corporel total, conduisant à un risque exagéré de calcifications dans les tissus mous et le cœur. Un nouvel agent, le sevelamer, est le premier chélateur du phosphate exempt de calcium. Il a été démontré que cet agent permet de contrôler efficacement les taux de phosphore chez des patients adultes présentant une ostéodystrophie rénale chronique ; il parait également diminuer l'incidence de calcifications coronariennes et aortiques, et semble avoir des effets bénéfiques sur le métabolisme lipidique et les phénomènes inflammatoires. Des données préliminaires suggèrent que le sevelamer peut être administré sans risque aux enfants [9]. Le risque d'induire une acidose métabolique chronique ne doit toutefois pas être négligé.

Calcimimétiques

Chez les patients dialysés, le traitement préventif de l'hyperparathyroïdie par le calcium et par les métabolites de la vitamine D est souvent compliqué par la survenue d'une hypercalcémie et d'une hyperphosphatémie. Les calcimimétiques, tels le chlorhydrate de cinacalcet, agissent au niveau des récepteurs sensibles au calcium (CaSR), diminuant les taux d'hormone parathyroïdienne sans augmenter la calcémie ou la phosphorémie. Des données expérimentales suggèrent que les calcimimétiques permettent de prévenir le risque d'hyperplasie parathyroïdienne et d'augmenter la masse osseuse [10]. Il est raisonnable de penser que les effets des calcimimétiques sur la sécrétion d'hormone parathyroïdienne sont les mêmes chez l'enfant et chez l'adulte. Il faut cependant se souvenir que les CaSR sont exprimés au niveau des cartilages de croissance, et que le rôle des CaSR dans la prolifération et la différentiation des chondrocytes n'est pas encore clairement défini.

Transplantation rénale

Le mycophenolate mofetil (MMF) est un immunosuppresseur dénué de néphrotoxicité. Lorsqu'il est utilisé en association avec des corticostéroïdes et des inhibiteurs des calcineurines, le MMF réduit l'incidence des rejets aigus et facilite la prise en charge des crises de rejet et de résistance au traitement. Des études pédiatriques récentes montrent que le MMF améliore la fonction rénale à court et long termes, et diminue la pression artérielle, probablement parce qu'il rend possible une réduction parallèle des inhibiteurs des calcineurines [11]. Une méta-analyse récente chez l'adulte indique que l'interruption des inhibiteurs des calcineurines améliore la filtration glomérulaire [12]. Des protocoles associant MMF et faibles doses d'inhibiteurs des calcineurines sont activement développés.

Insuffisance rénale aiguë chez le nouveau-né

Asphyxie et détresse respiratoire

Théophylline

Chez le nouveau-né, l'asphyxie périnatale est la cause principale d'insuffisance rénale aiguë. La suractivation de l'adénosine intrarénale semble jouer un rôle prépondérant dans la pathogenèse de la néphropathie vasomotrice hypoxique. Des études expérimentales ont démontré que la théophylline, un antagoniste non spécifique des récepteurs cellulaires de surface de l'adénosine, prévient la baisse du DFG induite par un stress hypoxémique [13]. Des études cliniques récentes confirment la prévention par la théophylline de la vasoconstriction rénale induite par l'hypoxie. Une amélioration significative de la créatininémie, de la clearance de la créatinine et de la balance hydrique a ainsi été observée chez des nouveau-nés souffrant d'asphyxie traités par la théophylline à titre prophylactique, confirmant ainsi les résultats décrits précédemment par Huet *et al.* [14]. La théophylline s'est également révélée bénéfique chez des nouveau-nés prématurés présentant une oligurie secondaire à un syndrome de détresse respiratoire (RDS) [15]. L'utilisation rationnelle de théophylline apparaît donc prometteuse chez les nouveau-nés oliguriques. Toutefois, l'innocuité du blocage des récepteurs de l'adénosine chez le sujet immature doit être démontrée avant que l'usage de la théophylline chez les nouveau-nés présentant une oligurie secondaire à des troubles respiratoires puisse être généralisé.

Reflux vésico-urétéral (RVU)

Un reflux vésico-urétéral est présent chez 1 % des nouveau-nés et des nourrissons et disparaît souvent spontanément avec les années. Un RVU se retrouve chez 50 % environ des enfants présentant une infection urinaire (IU) et a été considéré comme un risque majeur pour le développement de lésions parenchymateuses. Deux types de mesures préventives ont été proposés, à savoir :
– la correction chirurgicale ou endoscopique du RVU ;
– une prophylaxie antibiotique prolongée.

Une étude récente sur une période de 4 ans chez des enfants présentant un RVU bilatéral avec une néphropathie de reflux a démontré que le devenir de la fonction rénale était identique dans les deux types de traitement, médical ou chirurgical. Ces résultats ne confirment pas l'hypothèse selon laquelle la fonction rénale serait protégée par la correction du RVU chez des enfants présentant une néphropathie bilatérale [16]. Des lésions cicatricielles peuvent également se développer en l'absence de RVU démontrable. Plus nos connaissances progressent, plus il apparaît que lors de néphropathies de reflux sévères, les altérations parenchymateuses sont l'expression d'une dysplasie anténatale congénitale. Les études soigneuses d'Ismaili *et al.* ont apporté un éclairage nouveau sur la pathogenèse, le diagnostic clinique, les conséquences et la prise en charge du RVU. Ces observations sont résumées dans une excellente revue [17].

Investigation du RVU

La cysto-uréthrographie mictionnelle (CUM) reste la meilleure méthode pour visualiser la vessie et l'urètre, pour diagnostiquer la présence de valves urétrales postérieures, et pour mettre en évidence un RVU. Une méta-analyse effectuée par Gordon *et al.* [18] a démontré que le RVU primaire détecté par cystographie n'était cependant qu'un faible prédicteur d'une atteinte parenchymateuse et que l'absence de RVU à la CUM n'excluait pas une telle atteinte. Cette étude confirme l'impression selon laquelle le RVU primaire n'est pas suffisant à lui seul, ni même essentiel, pour le développement de lésions rénales parenchymateuses suite à la survenue d'une IU. Dès lors, la pratique d'une CUM doit être considérée au cas par cas, et décidée en fonction de la présence à l'examen ultrasonographique : a) d'une dilatation pyélique (> 7 mm chez le nouveau-né ; > 10 mm chez l'enfant) ; b) d'une dilatation pyélocaliciellen ou urétérale ; c) d'une mauvaise différentiation cortico-médullaire ; d) d'une dysplasie rénale ; e) d'un épaississement des parois pelviennes ou urétérales [17]. Une CUM de routine chez ces nouveau-nés asymptomatiques ne semble donc pas justifiée. Un examen ultrasonographique itératif est recommandé, et une CUM pratiquée uniquement lorsqu'apparaît une augmentation du diamètre pelvien, ou lorsque la dilatation pyélique est associée à des infections urinaires récidivantes.

À l'évidence, une CUM est indispensable lorsque la présence de valves urétrales postérieures est suspectée.

Correction chirurgicale et endoscopique du reflux

La réimplantation reste une intervention chirurgicale comportant des risques. Elle devrait donc être réservée aux situations où un traitement conservateur est contrindiqué. Il est intéressant de noter que des femmes enceintes ayant subi une réimplantation urétérale dans leur enfance présentent apparemment un plus grand risque de développer une hydronéphrose progressive, des infections urinaires, une hypertension artérielle, une insuffisance rénale, un avortement spontané ou une mort néonatale prématurée [19].

Le taux de succès du traitement endoscopique du RVU est considérablement plus faible que celui de la réimplantation chirurgicale. Ce taux est meilleur lors de RVU modéré. Une méta-analyse récente a démontré la disparition du reflux dans 79 % des cas de degrés I et II, 72 % des cas de degré III et 65 % des cas de degré IV, après une injection unique d'agents tels que téflon, collagène ou macroplastique [20]. La migration potentielle du produit injecté dans d'autres tissus, avec l'apparition d'une réaction granulomateuse sévère, est une source de préoccupation, les effets délétères de l'intervention étant probablement supérieurs aux avantages escomptés.

Prophylaxie antibiotique

L'utilisation d'une antibiothérapie prophylactique est basée sur l'hypothèse qu'un RVU stérile ne provoque pas de lésions cicatricielles et que la plupart des RVU disparaîtront spontanément avec le temps. Lorsqu'une prophylaxie est prescrite, elle doit couvrir la période comportant le plus de risques, à savoir les premières années de vie.

Le déficit néphronique

En 1992, DJ Barker a présenté une hypothèse fascinante sur l'origine fœtale des maladies cardiovasculaires apparaissant à l'âge adulte [21]. Cette hypothèse était basée sur l'observation d'une association entre le poids de naissance et la survenue tardive de maladies cardiovasculaires. Il existe en effet une corrélation significative entre le poids de naissance et la survenue tardive d'hypertension artérielle et d'insuffisance rénale chronique. Un petit poids de naissance est associé à une dimi-

nution congénitale du nombre de néphrons. Lorsqu'il est associé à un retard de croissance intra-utérin (RCIU), ce petit poids corrèle avec la survenue ultérieure d'insuffisance rénale et d'hypertension artérielle. De nombreux mécanismes ont été proposés pour expliquer l'origine fœtale des maladies rénales à l'âge adulte. Le déficit néphronique entraîne une adaptation compensatrice des néphrons existants, qui se manifeste par une hypertrophie et une hyperfiltration glomérulaires. Une hyperfiltration chronique, induite notamment par l'activation du système rénine-angiotensine-aldostérone (RAAS) provoque une sclérose glomérulaire, une hypertension artérielle, et conduit finalement à une insuffisance rénale terminale. Des études chez l'animal ont montré que différents facteurs perturbant l'environnement fœtal peuvent entraîner un déficit néphronique congénital, comme par exemple l'exposition fœtale à un régime maternel pauvre en protéines, une carence maternelle en vitamine A [22], ou en fer, une hyperglycémie maternelle, un excès d'hormones stéroïdiennes, ou l'administration à la mère gestante de gentamicine, d'ampicilline, ou de cyclosporine [23]. En sus de ces facteurs de risque, un rattrapage de poids trop rapide peut lui aussi augmenter le risque de maladie chronique à l'âge adulte. Des études prospectives récentes [24], bien planifiées, démontrent qu'à l'âge de 20 ans, un petit poids de naissance est :
– négativement associé à la concentration plasmatique de la créatinine ainsi qu'à l'albuminurie ;
– associé à une diminution de la fonction rénale, les valeurs les plus basses étant observées chez les adultes nés avec un petit poids de naissance et un RCIU.

Les risques de développer une insuffisance rénale associés à la prématurité et au RCIU justifient amplement un suivi à long terme des nouveau-nés présentant un petit poids de naissance. La recherche systématique d'une albuminurie, d'une protéinurie et d'une hypertension artérielle dans ce groupe de patients permettra de détecter précocement ceux qui parmi eux pourraient bénéficier d'une protection rénale active.

Néphroprotection

Une perte partielle de la masse néphronique, qu'elle soit aiguë ou chronique, est associée à une hypefiltration compensatrice par les néphrons épargnés. Le système rénine-angiotensine-aldostérone joue un rôle clé dans ce phénomène : en augmentant la pression intraglomérulaire, l'angiotensine II induit une hyperfiltration dans les néphrons résiduels. L'activation continue de l'angiotensine II produit des effets secondaires systémiques et rénaux, à savoir une hypertension artérielle, une prolifération des cellules mésangiales et une fibrose rénale interstitielle. Les inhibiteurs de l'enzyme de conversion de l'angiotensine (IECA) et/ou les antagonistes ses récepteurs AT1 de l'angiotensine II (ARA) ont un effet rénoprotecteur chez des patients présentant une néphropathie diabétique ou non-diabétique. Il faut noter cependant que ni les ICEAs ni les ARAs ne permettent de prévenir complètement la progression de la néphropathie. Ceci pourrait être dû au fait que ces agents n'entraînent pas de manière prévisible l'arrêt complet de la synthèse d'aldostérone. Ce phénomène dit « d'échappement de la synthèse d'aldostérone » pourrait être responsable d'une persistance d'effets potentiellement délétères de l'aldostérone [25].

Chez des enfants souffrant d'une néphropathie chronique progressive, l'administration pendant 6 mois d'un IECA, le ramipril, a permis d'améliorer clairement la protéinurie et l'hypertension artérielle [26]. Dans une autre étude plus récente d'une durée similaire et portant sur 10 enfants présentant une néphropathie chronique protéinurique, l'administration combinée d'IECAs et ARAs a significativement réduit la protéinurie, en comparaison à l'administration isolée de ces agents. Cette coadmistration d'un IECA et d'un ARA a eu pour effet de réduire l'hypertrophie ventriculaire gauche diagnostiquée par examen échocardiographique [27]. Des études cliniques pédiatriques portant sur les effets à long terme des IECAs ou des ARAs sur la progression des maladies rénales chroniques ne sont pas encore disponibles à ce jour.

Références

1. Gubler MC. Congenital and infantile nephrotic syndromes. *In* : Guignard JP, Gouyon JB, Simeoni U (eds). Développement rénal et programmation des maladies cardiovasculaires. Paris : Elsevier, 2005.
2. Cochat P, Liutkus A. Primary hyperoxaluria type 1 : still challenging. *Pediatr Nephrol* 2006 ; 8 : 1075-81.
3. Grubb A, Nyman U, Björk J, *et al.* Simple cystatin C-based prediction equations for glomerular filtration rate compared with the modification of diet in renal disease prediction equation for adults and the Schwartz and the Counahan-Barratt prediction equations for children. *Clin Chem* 2005 ; 51 : 1420-31.
4. Knight EL, Verhave JC, Spiegelman D, *et al.* Factors influencing serum systatin C levels other than renal function and the impact on renal function measurement. *Kidney Int* 2004 ; 65 : 1416-21.
5. Mendiluce A, Bustamante J, Martin D, *et al.* Cystatin C as a marker of renal function in kidney transplant patients. *Transplant Proc* 2005 ; 37 : 3844-7.
6. Martini S, Prevot A, Mosig D, *et al.* Glomerular filtration rate: measure creatinine and height rather that cystatin C! *Acta Paediatr* 2003 ; 92 : 1052-7.
7. Fujinaga S, Ohtomo Y, Umino D, *et al.* A prospective study on the use of mycophenolate mofetil in children with cyclosporin-dependent nephrotic syndrome. *Pediatr Nephrol* 2007 ; 22 : 71-6.
8. Schmitt CP, Nau B, Brummer C, *et al.* Increased injection pain with darbepoetin-alfa compared to epoetin-beta in paediatric dialysis patients. *Nephrol Dial Transplant* 2006 ; 21 : 3520-4.
9. Querfeld U. The therapeutic potential of novel phosphate binders. *Pediatr Nephrol* 2005 ; 20 : 389-92.
10. Goodman WG. Calcimimetics : a remedy for all problems of excess parathyroid hormone activity in chronic kidney disease. *Curr Opin Nephrol Hypertens* 2005 ; 14 : 355-60.

11. Kerecuk L, Taylor J, Clark G. Chronic allograft nephropathy and mycophenolate mofetil introduction in pediatric renal recipients. *Pediatr Nephrol* 2005 ; 20 : 1630-5.

12. Mulay AV, Hussain N, Fergusson D, Knoll GA. Calcineurin inhibitor withdrawal from sirolimus-based therapy in nkidney transplantation : a systematic review of randomized trials. *Am J Transplant* 2005 ; 5 : 1748-56.

13. Gouyon JB, Guignard JP. Theophylline prevents the hypoxemia-induced renal hemodynamic changes in rabbits. *Kidney Int* 1998 ; 33 : 1078-83.

14. Huet F, Semama D, Grimaldi M, et al. Effects of theophylline on renal insufficiency in neonates with respiratory distress syndrome. *Intensive Care Med* 1995 ; 21 : 511-4.

15. Cattarelli D, Spandrio M, Gasparoni A, et al. A randomized, double-blind, placebo-controlled trial of the effect of theophylline in prevention of vasomotor nephropathy in very preterm neonates with respiratory distress syndrome. *Arch Dis Child Fetal Neonatal* Ed 2006 ; 91 : F80-4.

16. Smellie JM, Barratt TM, Chantler C, et al. Medical versus surgical treatment in children with severe bilateral vesicouretic reflux and bilateral nephropathy : a randomised trial. *Lancet* 2001 ; 357 : 1329-33.

17. Ismaili K, Avni FE, Piepsz A, et al. Vesicoureteric reflux in children. *EAU-EBU Update Series* 2006 ; 4 : 129-40.

18. Gordon I, Barkovics M, Pindoria S, et al. Primary vesicouretic relux as a predictor of renal damage in children hospitalized with urinary tract infection: A systematic review and meta-analysis. *J Am Soc Nephrol* 2003 ; 14 : 739-44.

19. Bukowski TP, Betros GG, Aquilina JW, Perlmutter AD. Urinary tract infections and pregnancy in women who underwent antireflux surgery in childhood. *J Urol* 1998 ; 159 : 1286-9.

20. Elder JS, Peters CA, Arant BS, et al. Pediatric Vesicoureteral Reflux Guidelines Panel summary report on the management of primary vesicoureteral reflux in children. *J Urol* 1997 ; 157 : 1846-51.

21. Barker DJ. Fetal and Infant Origins of Adult Disease. London : BMJ Publisher, 1992.

22. Gilbert T, Merlet-Benichou C. Retinoids and nephron mass control. *Pediatr Nephrol* 2000 ; 14 : 1137-44.

23. Tendron-Franzin A, Gouyon JB, Guignard JP, et al. Long-term effects of in utero exposure to cyclosporin A on renal function in the rabbit. *J Am Nephrol Assoc* 2004 ; 15 : 2687-93.

24. Keijzer-Veen MG, Schrevel M, Finken MJ, et al. Microalbuminuria and lower filtration rate at young adult age in subjects born very prematurate and after intrauterine growth retardation. *J Am Soc Nephrol* 2005 ; 16 : 2762-8.

25. Aldigier JC, Kanjanbuch T, Ma LJ, et al. Remission of existing glomerulosclerosis by inhibition of aldosterone. *J Am Soc Nephrol* 2005 ; 16 : 3306-14.

26. Seeman T, Dusek J, Vondrak K, et al. Ramipril in the treatment of hypertension and proteinuria in children with chronic kidney diseases. *Am J Hypertens* 2004 ; 17 : 415-20.

27. Lubrano R, Soscia F, Elli M, et al. Renal and cardiovascular effects of angiotensin-converting enzyme inhibitor plus angiotensin II receptor antagonist therapy in children with proteinuria. *Pediatrics* 2006 ; 118 : e822-8.

Développements récents en pédopsychiatrie

Philippe JEAMMET

Chef de service de psychiatrie de l'adolescent et du jeune adulte,
Département de psychiatrie,
Institut Mutualiste Montsouris, Paris, France

Si l'évolution des connaissances peut paraître moins rapide et moins spectaculaire en pédopsychiatrie que dans d'autres domaines des pathologies de l'enfant et de l'adolescent, elle n'en est pas moins profonde. Nous choisirons pour l'illustrer trois champs d'études. Ces développements sont surtout le fait de l'apport des neurosciences, de la génétique et de la neuro-imagerie. Ces apports ne doivent pas faire oublier l'importance et la spécificité de leur inscription dans le développement de la personnalité et de son contexte relationnel qui en fait toute la complexité.

Vers une perspective intégrative de la compréhension étiopathogénique des troubles mentaux

Ces vingt dernières années ont vu un changement épistémologique radical avec un abandon de la perspective adultomorphe, jusque-là prédominante pour comprendre et traiter les questions de santé mentale de l'enfant, pour une perspective développementale. L'apport des connaissances sur comment se construit le psychisme peut contribuer à éclairer la pratique de l'adulte et l'enrichir de sa spécificité par une prise en compte de la complexité.

La perspective intégrative caractérise la compréhension étiopathogénique des phénomènes mentaux ainsi que les processus psychothérapeutiques [1]. Les approches théoriques, les disciplines scientifiques, les pratiques thérapeutiques ne sont plus vécues comme opposées les unes aux autres mais complémentaires : un même phénomène sera éclairé par les connaissances en génétique, en neurosciences, en biologie, en sciences psychologiques (cognitivisme, systémisme, psychologie développementale, traitement de l'information) et en sciences humaines (sociologie, anthropologie) favorisant *« la reconnaissance d'une causalité multiplie dans les désordres de l'enfance »* [2].

Il n'y a plus d'opposition inné/acquis, nature/nurturance mais interaction permanente entre la composante innée (génétique et intra-utérine) et les facteurs environnementaux postnatals. Les apports de la génétique moderne y contribuent.
Le début de la vie psychique n'est plus considéré comme intrapsychique mais d'abord interpersonnel puis secondairement intrapsychique surtout à partir de 2-3 ans. Le développement de la neurobiologie de l'interpersonnel [3] a montré que les expériences interactives interpersonnelles concourent à la constitution des câblages neuronaux, ainsi qu'au développement des capacités attentionnelles et de régulation émotionnelle. Ceci a des implications thérapeutiques résumées par Fonagy et al. [2] : *« la reconnaissance de l'importance des processus neurobiologiques a pour effet qu'à la fois les médicaments et les traitements psychosociaux peuvent accomplir des changements en agissant au niveau du cerveau »*.

L'être humain est replacé dans une perspective éthologique : que partageons-nous avec les autres espèces animales comme lois du vivant ? L'éthologie a apporté la notion de système motivationnel qui révolutionne la compréhension du développement et de ses troubles, compris dans une perspective évolutionniste. Les différentes composantes du fonctionnement humain peuvent être revues dans une perspective intégrative des systèmes motivationnels. Le concept de pulsion peut être replacé dans une perspective de système motivationnel (celui de l'hédonisme ou sexualité infantile) [4].

La complexité de l'étiopathogénie des troubles en santé mentale ne peut être actuellement comprise qu'en abandonnant les perspectives linéaires causalistes ou le modèle médical « défectologique ». Les nouveaux modèles du trouble en santé mentale sont davantage construits sur le modèle de la théorie des catastrophes : il y a une série de facteurs de risques et une absence de facteurs de protection à un moment plus ou moins sensible du développement. Les connaissances en psychologie développementale apportent dorénavant plusieurs certitudes :

– Un seul facteur de risque ne peut conduire à un trouble en santé mentale (à part les anomalies majeures génétiques comme dans l'autisme ou les retards mentaux).
– La compréhension du développement de l'être humain part des connaissances réelles actuelles sur le début de la vie grâce à l'explosion de techniques liées à la vidéo, l'informatique et non pas de la reconstruction, à partir d'adultes allant mal, de ce que serait le développement du bébé. Il n'y a plus de vue globale des fonctionnements et des relations mais des dimensions interactives plus ou moins synergétiques ou antagonistes (théorie de l'attachement, intersubjectivité).
– Les influences réciproques entre l'enfant et ceux qui l'élèvent sont importantes dans le développement d'éventuels troubles chez l'enfant ou de dysfonctionnements parentaux relationnels (illustration par exemple des troubles de la régulation dans la classification *zero to three*).
– On doit prendre en compte ce qu'un enfant est vraiment capable de faire selon son âge : développement des théories cognitives développementales [2].
– L'approche psychodynamique revalorisée mais nuancée par rapport à la théorie psychanalytique classique : celle-ci a apporté deux idées essentielles qui, à elles seules, justifient son importance : l'idée de phénomènes inconscients et l'idée que notre passé influence notre vie d'adulte.
– L'approche n'est plus structuraliste mais dimensionnelle, contextuelle et développementale. On comprend mieux le développement en psychiatrie des interfaces que sont la psychiatrie périnatale, la psychiatrie développementale ou précoce, celle de l'adolescent, qui toutes réclament la prise en compte de la complexité. L'approche développementale donne autant de poids au passé qu'au présent : « *la reconnaissance qu'insister uniquement sur les facteurs du passé (distaux) ou présents (proximaux) est tout autant inadéquate* » [2].
– L'importance du processus d'évaluation : la pratique moderne de la pédopsychiatrie demande une approche exhaustive des ressources et vulnérabilités de l'enfant [5] et repose sur des moyens différents (tests, évaluation standardisée, entretiens cliniques) répétés et prenant en compte le contexte, ce d'autant plus que l'enfant est jeune [2]. L'évaluation est simultanément diagnostique et thérapeutique : elle évalue ce qui vient de l'environnement, ce qui est lié à l'interaction, ce qui vient de l'enfant en tenant compte des résultats des recherches publiées sur des populations comparables. Il s'agit de repérer les processus biologiques, psychologiques et interpersonnels qui peuvent être sources de changement avec « *la reconnaissance qu'une évaluation adéquate doit inclure des informations à propos du développement et du savoir portant sur les populations d'enfants présentant des problèmes similaires (incidence, prévalence, facteurs biologiques, paramètres systémiques)* » [2].

Les classifications internationales adaptées à l'adulte sont revisitées en fonction des connaissances actuelles : un axe I contient les troubles syndromiques qui appartiennent à l'individu avec un poids peut-être plus important des facteurs biologiques et génétiques. Un axe II (axe de la personnalité) est lié aux questions des interactions interpersonnelles, aux axes somatiques, organiques, environnementaux stressants et du fonctionnement. On propose de rajouter un axe de l'alliance thérapeutique [6].

La compréhension des approches psychothérapeutiques se fait également de manière intégrative : « *l'engagement dans une trame théorique cohérente et fiable qui puisse guider une pratique qui lie les modèles de pathologie et le traitement au moins à un niveau conceptuel* » [2].

L'intérêt se porte actuellement sur l'importance des facteurs dits non spécifiques ou pan théoriques dans les prises en charge et sur la théorisation de ce qui se joue dans les facteurs non spécifiques des psychothérapies [7] et le concept d'alliance.
Ceci va de pair avec la compréhension plurithéorique de l'importance clé des processus interactifs entre le thérapeute et ses patients comme partie du traitement. C'est une nouvelle compréhension du transfert et contre transfert à la lumière des connaissances systémiques et des nouvelles théories du développement (intersubjectivité, attachement) [2, 8]. Le concept d'alliance thérapeutique développé chez l'adulte depuis les années 1970 s'est étendu à la pratique pédopsychiatrique depuis les années 1980 en raison du développement de la psychiatrie du bébé, de l'adolescent et de la psychiatrie périnatale. Ce développement est parti d'une position pragmatique : si on veut accéder aux enfants et les garder en soin, il faut que les parents supportent le soin. Il est lié aussi à la compréhension de plus en plus systémique des problèmes en santé mentale en pédopsychiatrie : on ne peut travailler sans les parents, on ne peut pas mettre l'enfant dans un conflit de loyauté, les parents sont aussi des partenaires du soin.

Les avancées scientifiques n'ont plus permis de considérer les parents comme seuls responsables des troubles de l'enfant comme cela était le cas jusqu'en 1980. La révolution dans la compréhension de l'autisme, la compréhension du transgénérationnel sont les paradigmes de ce changement. Les travaux de Fraiberg ont été pionniers [9].

La révolution de la théorie de l'attachement

Cette théorie développée par Bowlby [10] puis Ainsworth à partir des années 1970 est depuis les années 1990 source d'une révolution dans la compréhension du développement de l'enfant et de la pratique, analogue probablement à celle opérée par la psychanalyse au début du siècle.

Partant des observations sur la réaction d'un enfant à la séparation, Bowlby a été amené à se pencher sur la nature du lien mère-enfant. Les théories de la « pulsion secondaire » qui prévalaient au début de ses travaux dans les années 50, qu'elles soient issues de la psychanalyse ou de la théorie de l'apprentissage, décrivaient ce lien comme une conséquence des gratifications maternelles, au tout premier plan desquelles venait la nourriture. Dans ces conceptions, les seuls besoins primaires étaient ceux du corps.

Les travaux de Lorenz sur l'empreinte, qui mettaient ces théories en question, ont conduit Bowlby à faire l'hypothèse d'un comportement primaire d'attachement capable de lier l'enfant à sa mère. Pour Bowlby, la propension à établir des liens affectifs forts avec des personnes particulières est une composante fondamentale de la nature humaine.

Il a progressivement élaboré sa théorie cybernétique du comportement d'attachement qui vise à expliquer la constitution de l'ensemble des liens affectifs non seulement entre la mère et son enfant mais aussi entre adultes.

Si cette élaboration théorique doit beaucoup à la psychanalyse, formation initiale de Bowlby, et à l'éthologie, elle est d'un grand éclectisme et fait également intervenir des principes issus de la théorie cybernétique de la régulation ou théorie des systèmes, de la neurophysiologie, de la psychologie du développement et de la psychologie cognitive.

De l'éthologie vient l'idée que les comportements sociaux ont une dimension instinctive et que les relations peuvent être observées expérimentalement. De la théorie psychanalytique (relation d'objet) vient la notion d'un monde interne comportant des représentations de soi, des autres, et des relations entre les deux, ces représentations pouvant être déformées par l'immaturité ou les fantasmes.

Selon la théorie de l'attachement, le lien affectif de l'enfant à sa mère est le produit du comportement d'attachement. Le système comportemental d'attachement regroupe et organise l'ensemble des comportements de signal et d'approche dont le résultat est d'obtenir ou de maintenir une proximité vis-à-vis d'un individu donné, pour lequel il existe une préférence, le plus souvent la mère.

Ce système se développe dès les premiers mois de la vie. Dès sa naissance, le bébé est capable d'entrer dans une interaction sociale et montre du plaisir à le faire. Au cours des premières semaines, le bébé manifeste déjà un grand nombre des réactions constitutives de ce qui deviendra le comportement d'attachement. Toutefois ce comportement ne peut réellement s'organiser en système par rapport à une figure discriminée que lorsque l'enfant a la capacité cognitive de conserver sa mère à l'esprit lorsqu'elle est absente, capacité qui se développe au cours du deuxième semestre de la vie. C'est donc à partir de 9 mois environ que le système organisé se met en place pour atteindre une forme typique dans la deuxième année ; il est alors activé par le départ de la mère ou toute situation alarmante, et il cesse lorsque l'enfant peut voir, entendre ou toucher sa mère. Après l'âge de trois ans, l'activation de ce système comportemental est de moins en moins fréquente et sa désactivation est rendue possible par une gamme de plus en plus large de conditions, parfois purement symboliques.

Ainsi progressivement, plus que la présence effective de la figure d'attachement, ce sont les prévisions quant à la disponibilité de cette figure, intégrées sous forme de modèles de représentation, qui vont jouer le rôle principal.

Compte tenu de ces modifications, le comportement d'attachement et les liens auxquels il conduit vont persister tout au long de l'existence, sachant que surviennent également des changements concernant les figures vers lesquelles il est dirigé.

Ce sont les expériences vécues avec les figures d'attachement de la première enfance à l'adolescence qui déterminent la forme que prend le comportement d'attachement de l'adulte. Il s'agit là d'un point essentiel de la théorie de Bowlby, qui considère que le schème d'attachement qu'un individu développe pendant ses années d'immaturité est modelé par l'attitude de ses parents et a ensuite tendance à persister, devenant une qualité propre à cet individu, qui va imprégner ses nouvelles relations à autrui.
Deux grands types d'attachement ont été décrits :
– L'attachement « confiant » ou « sécure » où le contact avec la figure d'attachement se fait sans ambivalence rendant la séparation facile.
– L'attachement insécure qui a été subdivisé en :
    – attachement « évitant » (« *insecure-avoidants* ») : il existe un évitement de la figure d'attachement ; le contact n'est pas recherché mais n'est pas refusé non plus ;
    – attachement « ambivalent » (« *insecure-ambivalent* ») : le contact est recherché, mais il semble fui en même temps. L'enfant peut protester quand il est pris par la mère et protester quand il est posé. C'est pour ce type qu'on parle d'attachement anxieux ;
    – attachement « confus-désorganisé » (« *insecure-disorganized/disoriented* ») où dominent les postures d'appréhension, de confusion voire de dépression chez l'enfant.

Pour rendre compte de la persistance d'un schème d'attachement chez un individu donné, Bowlby a recours au concept de modèles internes opérants, de soi et des parents. Ce sont des modèles mentaux construits au cours des premières années à partir d'expériences réelles qui représentent les parents et le sujet lui-même, en fonction de l'image que ses parents ont de lui, et qui persistent par la suite même lorsque les circonstances sont modifiées.
Ainsi le comportement d'attachement aurait sa dynamique propre, distincte et d'une signification biologique égale au comportement alimentaire ou au comportement sexuel. Les liens auxquels il conduit existent pour eux-mêmes, certes en interaction avec ceux déterminés par le nourrissage et la sexualité, et ils ont, en tant que tels, une fonction vitale.

Ces systèmes comportementaux homéostatiques maintiennent en permanence la distance réelle ou symbolique par rapport à la figure d'attachement entre certaines limites. Tout décalage entre les instructions initiales et l'exécution en cours modifie le comportement en conséquence.

La plupart des émotions les plus intenses seraient en rapport avec le devenir de ce lien d'attachement. Son maintien ou son renouvellement entraîne joie et sensation de sécurité, sa rupture entraîne l'angoisse si elle est temporaire, le chagrin si elle est définitive.

Selon Bowlby, la pathologie résulte d'un cheminement déviant du comportement d'attachement, qui le plus souvent est à l'origine d'une activation trop fréquente de ce comportement, réalisant ce qu'il appelle l'attachement angoissé. Les formes les plus puissantes du comportement d'attachement provoquées par la menace de perte, dont l'équivalent est observé chez l'enfant au cours de la phase de protestation, surviennent alors fréquemment, réalisant des pathologies anxieuses telles que la phobie scolaire ou l'agoraphobie. L'équivalent de la phase de désespoir pourra de la même façon survenir de façon plus facile et plus prolongée chez certains sujets confrontés à des situations de perte dont le comportement d'attachement est perturbé du fait de déviations au cours du développement, réalisant dans ce cas un tableau de dépression.
Les modalités des liens d'attachement construits dans la petite enfance, tels qu'ils ont été décrits, sont stables en dehors de la survenue d'événements particuliers (deuils, traumatisme, rencontres, psychothérapie…) susceptibles de les remanier.

À partir de la fin de l'adolescence le système d'attachement jusque-là marqué par l'asymétrie des relations devient symétrique entre individus ayant atteint le même stade de développement psychologique. Les liens d'attachement s'établissent alors dans la réciprocité.

Au sein de ces relations adultes, des différences importantes existent entre les relations amicales qui représentent des figures d'attachement auxiliaires et le partenaire amoureux qui représente, après un certain temps de relation qui semble se situer autour de deux ou trois ans, la figure d'attachement principale.
Dans la plupart des cas, le partenaire sexuel joue donc le rôle de la figure d'attachement principale à l'âge adulte et prend la place des parents de l'enfance.

Plus qu'une théorie globale du fonctionnement psychique, la théorie de l'attachement représente un cadre conceptuel qui porte sur les relations et plus précisément sur les aspects de la relation qui touchent aux besoins de sécurité. C'est par essence une théorie spatiale : quand je suis près de celui ou celle auquel je suis attaché, je me sens bien ; quand je suis loin je me sens anxieux ou triste. L'attachement passe par la vue, l'ouïe, le toucher, qui procurent l'apaisement, le sentiment de sécurité, ces derniers permettant ensuite de s'éloigner pour explorer.

Vers une continuité entre troubles psychiatriques de l'enfance et pathologies de l'adulte

Le développement des études génétiques et la neurobiologie plaident en faveur d'une continuité des troubles en particulier pour les deux pathologies centrales que représentent les troubles de l'humeur et le spectre des troubles schizophréniques.

La problématique s'est progressivement déplacée de la reconnaissance ou non du trouble au cours de l'enfance vers celle du mode d'expression spécifique ou non à cet âge. Ainsi la question d'éventuelles particularités de ces pathologies à cet âge se pose : doit-on parler de troubles *de* l'enfance ou de troubles *dès* l'enfance ? La difficulté majeure posée aujourd'hui réside dans la possibilité d'opérationnaliser des critères valides et reconnus du trouble. Ainsi l'identification d'un trouble chez l'enfant implique de différencier cette entité des expériences habituelles liées au développement et de séparer ces troubles des autres pathologies de cet âge.
Les travaux les plus récents montrent que le trouble dépressif majeur est une maladie familiale récurrente qui interfère significativement avec le développement émotionnel et cognitif normal de l'enfant. Il est associé avec un risque accru de tentatives de suicide, avec d'autres troubles psychiatriques tels que la toxicomanie et les problèmes de comportement, un fonctionnement psychosocial et scolaire difficile : sa survenue dans l'enfance et l'adolescence accroît fortement d'une part le risque d'épisodes dépressifs et récurrents et d'autre part de difficultés psychosociales à l'âge adulte [11-13]. La prévalence de ce trouble chez les enfants et les adolescents est évaluée entre 2 et 6 % avec un accroissement de fréquence avec l'âge. L'ensemble des études actuelles montre que le risque de développer un trouble de l'humeur et de le développer de plus en plus tôt s'accroît avec les enfants nés récemment.
Plus de 50 % des adultes avec un trouble dépressif majeur rapportent que leur dépression a commencé pendant l'enfance. Des études cliniques et sur des groupes de population ont également montré que la survenue d'un syndrome dépressif majeur à l'adolescence est un risque majeur de dépression chez l'adulte et qu'il est associé avec un risque de morbidité psychiatrique, de difficultés de personnalité, de problèmes de travail, de mauvais résultats scolaires et d'un taux de mortalité par suicide élevé chez l'adulte [13-18].

Les facteurs familiaux qui influencent la survenue et l'évolution du trouble peuvent être génétiques ou non génétiques. Plusieurs études montrent une influence de facteurs génétiques sur l'âge de début et les rechutes. Les facteurs environnementaux familiaux tels que la dépression parentale avec ses répercussions sur le style de gestion du stress, les difficultés de faire face aux tâches parentales, l'irritabilité et l'instabilité du comportement, les difficultés économiques liées à l'incapacité à travailler accroissent le risque de dépression [19-21]. Il en est de même de l'exposition

aux événements négatifs comme les expériences de deuils et d'abandon, les abus sexuels, les conflits permanents.
De même, les études longitudinales des enfants et adolescents déprimés ont montré que 5 à 30 % d'entre eux développeront par la suite des épisodes de manie ou d'hypomanie.

Une histoire familiale de troubles de l'humeur en particulier de type récurrent chez les apparentés au 1er degré et une histoire antérieure des troubles de l'humeur chez l'enfant sont des facteurs de risque concernant la précocité, la durée et la récurrence du syndrome dépressif majeur.

Le syndrome dépressif majeur ayant une forte propension à la récurrence, il apparaît important que le traitement soit suffisamment long pour éviter les rechutes. Les études sur les traitements à court terme ont montré le risque élevé de rechutes après arrêt du traitement psychothérapique ou antidépresseur [22]. Les études contrôlées ou naturalistiques sur la durée du traitement ont montré, quant à la fréquence des rechutes, la supériorité des traitements à long terme comparés aux traitements brefs.

La réactualisation du trouble schizophrénique précoce illustre également l'évolution en matière de reconnaissance des pathologies chez l'enfant. Plus que la question absolue de l'existence d'un tel trouble, cette démarche met en lumière la diversité des processus pathologiques du développement et leur différenciation est d'autant plus importante que les retombées pourraient s'exprimer en termes de mécanismes de vulnérabilité plus qu'en termes de conduites thérapeutiques.
Les antécédents familiaux de schizophrénie et de troubles schizophréniformes sont fréquents dans les familles d'enfants schizophrènes, de même que les troubles affectifs.

Comme dans les formes adultes, les présentations cliniques sont nombreuses. Les formes très précoces ont généralement un début insidieux alors qu'à l'adolescence les débuts aigus sont plus fréquents. La symptomatologie se distingue entre symptômes positifs et négatifs comme dans les formes adultes. Le comportement désorganisé pourrait constituer un troisième groupe indépendant fait de signes associant la désorganisation du discours, la bizarrerie du comportement avec une faible capacité d'attention. Les hallucinations, le trouble du cours de la pensée et les affects émoussés sont fréquemment rapportés, mais les délires systématisés et les formes catatoniques sont plus rares. Chez le jeune enfant schizophrène, l'origine des hallucinations est fréquemment un animal et quand une voix est identifiée elle est souvent attribuée à un proche. Pour faciliter la reconnaissance de vraies hallucinations, il peut être important de demander à l'enfant s'il peut faire venir et disparaître ses voix à volonté. Les enfants schizophrènes rapportent fréquemment des hallucinations visuelles (30 % des cas) ou tactiles (17 %), qui accompagnent généralement des hallucinations auditives (présentes dans 80 % des cas), mais qui doivent faire rechercher une étiologie organique. Chez l'adolescent, les hallucinations sont qualitativement proches de celles décrites par les adultes. Les délires sont assez peu fréquents dans les formes précoces de schizophrénie (environ 60 % des cas) et ils deviennent plus complexes, élaborés et fixés avec l'âge. Avant l'âge de 10 ans, les thèmes concernent la perte de l'identité (les enfants s'identifient comme étant d'autres personnes, des animaux ou des objets) et des peurs diffuses et irrationnelles, souvent d'origine cosmique. Entre 10 et 14 ans, les thèmes se rapprochent de ceux des formes adultes avec persécution, transformation corporelle, thèmes religieux…

Il semble que la fréquence des symptômes positifs augmente avec l'âge et qu'ils soient plus fréquents quand le QI est supérieur à 85, tandis que les symptomatologies négatives seraient associées avec les lésions cérébrales et seraient plus fréquentes dans les débuts très précoces et en fin d'adolescence.

Les modes de communication sont particuliers chez ces enfants. En comparaison d'enfants sains, les enfants schizophrènes présentent davantage de ruptures associatives, de pensées illogiques et de difficultés d'élocution. Cependant, il importe de tenir compte du niveau du développement de l'enfant.

Les antécédents prémorbides les plus fréquemment retrouvés sont l'isolement et le repli, les comportements perturbateurs, les difficultés de langage, motrices, scolaires, dans les relations sociales avec les pairs et les retards développementaux. Les altérations prémorbides semblent plus fréquentes dans les formes à début prépubertaire que dans celles à début plus tardif.

Il est établi que des stress psychosociaux, notamment la nature de l'expression des émotions au sein de la famille, influencent le début ou la récidive des épisodes aigus. Des déficits de communication sont fréquemment retrouvés chez les familles d'enfants schizophrènes, ce qui est davantage témoin de vulnérabilités génétiques que facteur causal en soi. Le rôle des facteurs socioéconomiques est discuté, sans valeur probante. Les antécédents familiaux de schizophrénie et de troubles schizophréniformes sont fréquents dans les familles d'enfants schizophrènes, de même que les troubles affectifs.

Au total, il semble que les formes précoces et très précoces de schizophrénies ne diffèrent que par des aspects quantitatifs et développementaux, et que la continuité des troubles soit la règle entre ces formes et avec les formes adultes.

En terme de conclusion, la réactualisation du trouble schizophrénique précoce illustre l'évolution en matière de reconnaissance des pathologies chez l'enfant. Plus que la question absolue de l'existence d'un tel trouble, cette démarche met en lumière la diversité des processus pathologiques du développement, et leur différenciation est d'autant plus importante que les retombées pourraient s'exprimer davantage en termes de mécanismes et de vulnérabilité qu'en termes de conduites thérapeutiques. L'intérêt d'une recherche sur le sujet est important pour mieux comprendre la schizophrénie, ses facteurs de risques, et ses modes de début, les interventions préventives et thérapeutiques possibles, ainsi que pour développer une réelle collaboration entre psychiatres d'enfants et psychiatres d'adultes autour des continuités et discontinuités des pathologies schizophréniques.

Références

1. Holmes J. Attachment theory : a biological basis for psychotherapy ? *Br J Psychiatry* 1993 ; 163 : 430-438.
2. Fonagy P, Target M, Cottrell D, et al. *What works for whom? A critical review of treatments for children and adolescents.* New York : The Guildford Press, 2002.
3. Shore A. Attachment and the regulation of the right brain. *Attachment & Human Development* 2000 ; 2 : 23-47.
4. Lichtenberg JD. Écouter, comprendre et interpréter. Réflexions sur la complexité. *Psychothérapies* 2004 ; 24 : 55-72.
5 Zeanah C. ed. *Handbook of Infant Mental Health.* New York : Guildford Press, 2000.
6. Guedeney N, Guedeney A, Rabouam C, et al. L'utilisation de la classification diagnostique Zero to Three à partir d'une observation. *Prisme* 2000 ; 33 : 80-91.
7. Cramer B. Can therapists learn from psychotherapy research. In : Von Klitzing K, Tyson P, Burgin D. (eds) *Psychoanalysis in childhood and adolescence.* Basel : Karger, 2000 ; 12-22.
8. Holmes J. *The search for a secure base. Attachment theory and psychotherapy.* New York : Routledge, 2001.
9. Fraiberg S. *Clinical studies of infant mental health. The first year of life.* London : Tavistock Publications, 1980.
10. Bowlby J. *A secure base.* New York : Basic Books, 1988.
11. Birmaher B, Ryan ND, Williamson DE, et al. Childhood and adolescent depression. A review of the past ten years. Part I, *J Am Acad Child Adolesc Psychiatry* 1996 ; 35 : 1427-39.
12. Fombonne E, Wostear G, Cooper V et al., The Maudsley long term follow-up of chills and adolescent depression. Suicidality, criminality and social dysfunction in adulthood. *Br J Psychiatry* 2001 ; 179 : 218-23.
13. Lewinsohn PM, Allen NB, Seeley JR, et al, First onset versus recurrence of depression: Differential processes of psychosocial risk. *J Abnorm Psychol* 1999 ; 108 : 483-89.
14. Harrington R, Fudge H, Rutter M et al. Adult outcomes of child and adolescent depression. I Psychiatric status. *Arch General Psychiatry* 1990 ; 47 : 465-73.
15. Rao U, Dahl RE, Ryan ND et al, Unipolar depression in adolescents: Clinical outcome in adulthood. *J Am Acad Child Adolesc Psychiatry* 1995 ; 34 : 566-78.
16. Rueter MA, Scaramella L, Wallace LE et al. First onset of depressive symptoms or anxiety disorder predicted by the longitudinal course of internalizing symptoms and parent-adolescent disagreements. *Arch Gen Psychiatry* 1999 ; 56 : 726-32.
17. Bardone AM, Moffitt TE, Caspi A, et al. Adult mental health and social outcomes of adolescent girls with depression and conduct disorder. *Dev Psychopathol* 1996 ; 8 : 811-29.
18. Rao U, Hammen C, Daley SE, et al. Continuity of depression during the transition to adulthood: A 5-year longitudinal study of women. *J Am Acad Child Adolesc Psychiatry* 1999 ; 38 : 908-15.
19. Klein DN, Lewinsohn PM, Seeley Jr, et al. A family study of major depressive disorder in a community sample of adolescents. *Arch General Psychiatry* 2001 ; 58 : 13-20.
20. Wickramaratne PJ, Weissman MM. Onset of psychopathology in offspring by developmental phase and parental depression. *J Am Acad Child Adolesc Psychiatry* 1998 ; 37 : 933-42.

21. Birmaher B, Brent DA, Kolko D, *et al.* Clinical outcome after short-term psychotherapy for adolescents with major depressive disorder. *Arch Gen Psychiatry* 2000 ; 57 : 29-36.
22. Brent DA, Holder D, Kolko D, *et al.* A clinical psychotherapy trial for adolescent depression comparing cognitive, family and supportive therapy. *Arch General Psychiatry* 1997 ; 54 : 877-85.

Les progrès récents en néonatalogie

Hugo LAGERCRANTZ*

Karolinska Institute, Hôpital pour Enfants Astrid Lindgren, Stockholm, Suède

La néonatalogie fait partie des quelques domaines de la médecine dans lesquels les progrès au cours des cinquante dernières années ont été particulièrement importants. Ces progrès sont illustrés par la baisse de la mortalité infantile survenue dans pratiquement tous les pays du monde et par l'augmentation significative de la survie des prématurés notée surtout dans les pays occidentaux. Certaines de ces avancées sont étroitement liées à des découvertes qui ont valu à leurs auteurs un prix Nobel de médecine.

Nobel 1906 et 1935 : les bases du développement cérébral

La compréhension du développement cérébral a bénéficié des travaux de Ramon y Cajal et Camillo Golgi sur la structure du système nerveux et de Hans Spemman sur l'induction embryonnaire et la morphogenèse, récompensés par un prix Nobel attri-

* Rédaction : Catherine Faber, d'après la communication de Hugo Lagercrantz au Colloque Charles Nicolle de Rouen.

bué, respectivement, en 1906 et en 1935. Les recherches menées au cours des dernières années ont permis d'identifier les facteurs impliqués dans ce phénomène, concernant en particulier la différentiation de l'ectoderme en tissu nerveux embryonnaire (induction neurale) et son blocage par le BMP (*brain morphogenic factor*). Les antagonistes du BMP, comme la noggine ou la follistatine, qui peuvent correspondre à l'organisateur de Spemann, participent à l'induction neurale [1].

Des données récentes suggèrent également que la migration neuronale est un évènement majeur de l'ontogenèse cérébrale. Les anomalies de cette migration peuvent jouer un rôle dans la genèse de l'autisme et de la schizophrénie. Certains travaux suggèrent que les infections virales au cours de la grossesse sont une cause non génétique majeure de l'autisme et, par ailleurs, augmentent le risque de schizophrénie, en particulier chez les enfants appartenant à des familles atteintes. Les fœtus exposés à un stress important semblent également plus à risque de schizophrénie. Les troubles de l'expression des molécules du complexe majeur d'histocompatibilité (CMH) sont un des mécanismes évoqués pour expliquer ces observations [2]. On sait en effet que les molécules CMH de classe 1 sont normalement exprimées par les neurones et jouent un rôle important dans le câblage du réseau neuronal [3].

Du Nobel 1981 aux soins de développement

En permettant d'élucider la physiopathologie de l'amblyopie, les travaux sur les mécanismes de transmission de l'information dans le système visuel de David Hubel, Torsten Wiesel et Roger Sperry, récipiendaires du Nobel de médecine 1981, ont eu un impact important en néonatalogie. Ils ont montré, chez l'animal, que l'élimination de l'activité rétinienne par obstruction d'un œil durant une période critique de quelques semaines après la naissance perturbe la structure des colonnes de dominance oculaire. Celle-ci résulte de la séparation des axones du noyau du corps géniculé latéral en colonnes spécifiquement liées à un œil dans le cortex visuel primaire. Ce processus implique la formation, l'élimination et la réorganisation des connexions synaptiques individuelles [4]. Son blocage par des toxines, comme la tétrodotoxine, entraîne une cécité.

À l'heure actuelle, l'impact clinique de ces données expérimentales reste du domaine de l'hypothèse. Chez les prématurés, les surstimulations engendrées par l'environnement lumineux et sonore des services de néonatalogie ainsi que le grand nombre de gestes invasifs ou inconfortables qu'ils subissent pourraient affecter l'induction et la connexion des neurones. Quelques études ont montré que les anciens prématurés ont un risque accru de syndrome d'hyperactivité avec déficit de l'attention (SHDA), d'anxiété, de phobies et de troubles cognitifs [5], y compris ceux qui ne présentent pas de lésions sévères du système nerveux central.

Un programme de développement a été conçu dans le but de prévenir ces séquelles neuropsychologiques : le NIDCAP (*Newborn individualized developmental care and assessment program*) fondé sur la réduction des surstimulations externes et des actes invasifs, avec la réalisation des soins en fonction de l'observation du bébé, et la participation des parents. D'après une étude par IRM en tenseurs de diffusion, comparés aux soins conventionnels, ces soins de développement semblent améliorer la myélinisation [6]. Une amélioration de l'évolution à long terme (3 ans) a également été constatée chez les enfants qui ont bénéficié du NIDCAP. Comme le suggèrent plusieurs études, ces résultats pourraient avoir un fondement biologique impliquant les récepteurs des glucocorticoïdes et la sérotonine.

Nobel 1979 et 2003 : l'imagerie cérébrale

Deux techniques d'imagerie récentes ont révolutionné la médecine néonatale : le scanner et l'IRM, dont la mise au point et le développement ont permis à leurs auteurs de remporter les prix Nobel de médecine 1979 (Allan Cormack et Geoffrey Hounsfield) et 1983 (Paul Lauterbur et Peter Mansfield).

Grâce au scanner cérébral, on s'est rendu compte de la fréquence des hémorragies intraventriculaires chez les prématurés [7]. Cet examen et l'IRM ont aussi permis de découvrir que les très grands prématurés présentent souvent des lésions de la substance blanche [8, 9]. Les tenseurs de diffusion permettent une étude de la myélinisation.

Les techniques de résonance magnétique peuvent être utilisées comme un outil de suivi à long terme. Avec cette imagerie, des équipes ont mis en évidence une diminution significative du volume de certaines zones cérébrales chez les anciens prématurés adolescents [5] et une anisotropie basse indiquant un trouble de la myélinisation à l'âge de 11 ans [10].

Par ailleurs, les réactions aux stimuli sensoriels comme la douleur ont été étudiées par IRM fonctionnelle. Cet examen étant difficile à répéter chez les bébés, les données sur ce sujet sont issues essentiellement d'études réalisées chez des adultes et des enfants plus grands. Des informations intéressantes ont toutefois été mises en évidence chez le nouveau-né par d'autres techniques comme la spectroscopie proche infrarouge qui permet une mesure semiquantitative du flux sanguin au niveau des aires sensorielles. Deux équipes indépendantes ont ainsi montré que le cortex sensoriel des prématurés est activé par la douleur [11, 12].

Nobel 1936, 1970 et 1982 : les neurotransmetteurs chimiques

Trois prix Nobel ont été attribués aux auteurs de découvertes sur la neurotransmission chimique.

En 1936, Henry Dale et Otto Loewi ont été récompensés pour leurs travaux sur la transmission chimique des impulsions nerveuses et en 1970 Bernard Katz, Ulf von Euler et Julius Axelrod l'ont été pour leurs découvertes sur les transmetteurs humoraux dans les terminaisons nerveuses et les mécanismes de leur stockage, de leur libération et de leur inactivation. Les catécholamines, transmetteurs chimiques les plus importants en néonatalogie, jouent probablement un rôle dans l'adaptation néonatale, comme le suggère la différence des taux plasmatiques de noradrénaline et d'adrénaline mise en évidence chez le fœtus et le nouveau-né selon le mode d'accouchement. Très élevés lors de l'accouchement par voie basse, ces taux sont bas si celui-ci se fait par césarienne. Certains troubles comme le poumon de choc et l'hypoglycémie pourraient être liés à une élévation insuffisante des catécholamines [13].

La dopamine est largement utilisée pour traiter l'hypotension. Une relation entre des perturbations du *turnover* de la monoamine oxydase – enzyme métabolisant les catécholamines – et le développement du SHDA et d'autres troubles psychiatriques a été évoquée. Il existe quelques arguments indiquant que l'hypoxie fœtale peut entraîner des perturbations de ce *turnover* à l'âge adulte (Peyronnet). Cette voie de recherche sur la programmation développementale s'avère des plus prometteuses [14].
En 1982, Sune Bergström, Bengt Samuelson et John Vane ont reçu le Nobel de médecine et de physiologie pour leurs travaux sur les prostaglandines (PG) et les substances biologiques actives liées aux PG, qui ont eu un impact majeur en médecine reproductive et néonatale. Outre leur rôle dans la persistance du canal artériel – dont le traitement repose sur des antagonistes des PG comme l'indométacine et l'ibuprofène –, les PG semblent être importantes dans la suppression des mouvements respiratoires fœtaux. Un inhibiteur placentaire de la respiration a été identifié comme une PG [15, 16]. Des études récentes ont montré que l'indométacine – un inhibiteur de la synthèse des PG – a un effet neuroprotecteur à long terme, en particulier chez les garçons [17].

Autre transmetteur d'intérêt en néonatalogie : l'oxyde nitrique (NO). Le NO qui semble impliqué dans la dilatation des artères pulmonaires à la naissance [18], est devenu un traitement de choix dans l'hypertension artérielle pulmonaire persistante du nouveau-né et la circulation fœtale persistante, et réduit significativement le besoin de circulation extracorporelle. Le NO est également une molécule prometteuse pour la prévention de la dysplasie bronchopulmonaire : il diminue l'accumulation des neutrophiles pulmonaires et, par conséquent, la cascade inflammatoire qui conduit au développement de cette pathologie [19]. Enfin, le NO pourrait avoir un effet neuroprotecteur.

Références

1. Jessell TM, Sanes JR. The decade of the developing brain. *Current opinion in neurobiology* 2000 ; 10 : 599-611.
2. Boulanger LM, Shatz CJ. Immune signalling in neural development, synaptic plasticity and disease. *Nat Rev Neurosci* 2004 ; 5 : 521-31.
3. Belmonte MK, Allen G, Beckel-Mitchener A, *et al.* Autism and abnormal development of brain connectivity. *J Neurosci* 2004 ; 24 : 9228-31.
4. Katz LC, Shatz CJ. Synaptic activity and the construction of cortical circuits. *Science* 1996 ; 274 : 1133-8.
5. Ment LR, Vohr B, Allan W, *et al.* Change in cognitive function over time in very low-birth-weight infants. *JAMA* 2003 ; 289 : 705-11.
6. Als H, Duffy FH, McAnulty GB, *et al.* Early experience alters brain function and structure. *Pediatrics* 2004 ; 113 : 846-57.
7. Fitzhardinge PM, Flodmark O, Fitz CR, Ashby S. The prognostic value of computed tomography of the brain in asphyxiated premature infants. *J Pediatr* 1982 ; 100 : 476-81.
8. Huppi PS. Immature white matter lesions in the premature infant. *J Pediatr.* 2004 ; 145 : 575-8.
9. Inder TE, Warfield SK, Wang H, Huppi PS et al. Abnormal cerebral structure is present at term in premature infants. *Pediatrics* 2005 ; 115 : 286-94.
10. Nagy Z, Westerberg H, Skare S, Andersson JL et al. Preterm children have disturbances of white matter at 11 years of age as shown by diffusion tensor imaging. *Pediatr Res* 2003 ; 54 : 672-9.
11. Fitzgerald M, Walker S. Infant pain traces. *Pain* 2006 ; 125 : 204-5.
12. Bartocci M, Bergqvist LL, Lagercrantz H, Anand KJ. Pain activates cortical areas in the preterm newborn brain. *Pain* 2006 ; 122 : 109-17.
13. Lagercrantz H, Nilsson E, Redham I, Hjemdahl P. Plasma catecholamines following nursing procedures in a neonatal ward. *Early Hum Dev* 1986 ; 14 : 61-5.
14. Barker DJ. Fetal origins of cardiovascular disease. *Ann Med* 1999 ; 31 : 3-6.
15. Rigatto H. Regulation of fetal breathing. *Reprod Fertil Dev* 1996 ; 8 : 23-33.
16. Alvaro RE, Hasan SU, Chemtob S, Qurashi M et al. Prostaglandins are responsible for the inhibition of breathing observed with a placental extract in fetal sheep. *Respir Physiol Neurobiol* 2004 ; 144 : 35-44.
17. Ment LR, Vohr BR, Makuch RW, Westerveld M et al. Prevention of intraventricular hemorrhage by indomethacin in male preterm infants. *J Pediatr* 2004 ; 145 : 832-4.
18. Rairigh RL, Parker TA, Ivy DD, *et al.* Role of inducible nitric oxide synthase in the pulmonary vascular response to birth-related stimuli in the ovine fetus. *Circ Res* 2001 ; 88 : 721-6.
19. Kinsella JP. Inhaled nitric oxide therapy in premature newborn. *Curr Opin Pediatr* 2006 ; 18 : 107-111.

Présent et futur en vaccinologie

Stanley PLOTKIN*

Université de Pennsylvanie, Philadelphia, PA, USA

La vaccination a aujourd'hui deux cents ans.

L'histoire des vaccins débute avec les travaux de Jenner qui observe que la vaccination protège contre la variole. Mais ce sont les travaux de Pasteur dans les années 1880 qui définissent le principe d'action de la vaccination et inaugurent véritablement la vaccinologie avec la mise au point du premier vaccin humain contre la rage. Dans la première partie du 20e siècle, on développe de nouvelles méthodes d'atténuation de la virulence par passage sur des animaux, des œufs ou *in vitro* qui conduisent à la mise au point du vaccin BCG, du vaccin contre la fièvre jaune… Après la deuxième guerre mondiale de nombreux autres vaccins vivants atténués seront mis au point : rougeole, poliomyélite, oreillons, plus tard varicelle, rubéole, grippe. Parallèlement sont élaborés des vaccins inactivés : vaccin contre la typhoïde, contre le choléra, l'hépatite A, etc. Les recherches sur les anatoxines dans les années 20 ont conduit au développement des vaccins diphtérie et tétanos. Les techniques de fragmentation des organismes sont utilisées pour l'élaboration des vaccins contre l'anthrax, la rage. D'autres progrès encore ont été accomplis avec les travaux sur la capsule polysaccharidique de certaines bactéries qui ont abouti au développement de vaccins polysaccharidiques comme le vaccin antipneumococcique. La possibilité également d'individualiser les protéines a permis l'élaboration du vaccin coqueluche acellulaire ou encore du premier vaccin contre l'hépatite B. Enfin le

---

* Rédaction : Hélène Collignon, d'après la communication de Stanley Plotkin au Colloque Charles Nicolle de Rouen.
Article publié préalablement dans *Médecine et Enfance*.

procédé de conjugaison du polysaccharide de capsule avec une protéine porteuse a abouti à la mise au point de vaccins contre l'*Haemophilus influenzae B*, le pneumocoque et le méningocoque C, efficaces dès les premiers mois de vie.

Grâce aux progrès accomplis par la vaccination au cours de ces deux siècles, on a assisté à une disparition des grands fléaux dans les pays développés et à une forte réduction de la mortalité par infection dans les pays en voie de développement, bien qu'il reste encore beaucoup à faire pour que tous les enfants de ces pays bénéficient des vaccins disponibles. Ces progrès ont eu, bien entendu, des répercussions économiques importantes, le coût des vaccins et de la vaccination étant moindre que ceux, directs et indirects, générés par les maladies.

Les leçons de la vaccinologie

Première leçon : le système immunitaire est redondant

Néanmoins presque tous les vaccins actuels reposent sur les anticorps sériques et muqueux qui bloquent l'infection, la bactériémie ou la virémie. La seule exception concerne la tuberculose où le vaccin agit en réduisant la réplication du bacille dans les cellules macrophages.

On dispose aujourd'hui d'autres vaccins qui agissent sur l'immunité cellulaire. C'est le cas du vaccin varicelle qui a permis, aux États Unis où il est très largement utilisé, de réduire l'incidence de la maladie de 80 %. Le virus de la varicelle est responsable de deux maladies, la varicelle elle-même et le zona qui résulte de la réactivation du virus varicelle dans les neurones. Cette réactivation s'explique par la diminution de l'immunité cellulaire contre la varicelle après l'âge de 40 ans. À l'heure actuelle, le vaccin varicelle est utilisé chez les adultes pour relancer l'immunité cellulaire, réactiver les cellules T et réduire ainsi les conséquences de la réactivation du virus dans les neurones. Une vaste étude menée aux États Unis a montré que le vaccin varicelle (Zostavax®) permettait, chez l'adulte, de réduire d'environ 50 % la réactivation du virus et de diminuer également de deux tiers les neuralgies du zona. L'utilisation de ce vaccin chez les adultes de 60-65 ans permettrait de prévenir un grand nombre de zonas et de réduire significativement la gêne occasionnée par la maladie.

Deuxième leçon : l'immunité est plus forte vis-à-vis de la maladie que vis-à-vis de l'infection

Ceci est bien illustré par l'infection à rotavirus. Le rotavirus a un génome fragmenté (onze fragments d'ARN dans le noyau). Il porte sur sa surface deux protéines, les protéines P et G, qui sont particulièrement importantes car elles induisent la formation d'anticorps neutralisants permettant la protection contre les formes sévères de l'infection. Un rotavirus bovin a été isolé dans les années 80. Cette souche bovine est naturellement atténuée pour l'homme. Par un processus dit de réassortiment, on a pu infecter cette souche bovine avec une souche humaine et sélectionner ensuite les souches contenant dix fragments du virus bovin atténué et un fragment du virus humain produisant les protéines P et G. C'est ainsi qu'a été élaboré un vaccin pentavalent contenant les quatre protéines G et la protéine P les plus communément présentes dans le rotavirus humain. La protection conférée par ce vaccin s'exerce davantage contre la maladie que contre l'infection. Ainsi, dans une étude comparant des sujets vaccinés et des sujets témoins, le taux d'infection par le rotavirus a été équivalent dans les deux groupes. En revanche il n'y a eu aucun malade parmi les vaccinés alors qu'on en a dénombré 21 % dans le groupe témoin. Les résultats récents concernant ce vaccin qui a eu un développement élargi montrent qu'il donne une protection de 98 % contre les gastroentérites sévères et de 74 % contre toutes les formes de la maladie.

Troisième leçon : l'immunité naturelle est généralement meilleure que l'immunité vaccinale

C'est ce qu'atteste parfaitement une expérience réalisée il y a quelques années avec le cytomégalovirus, principale cause infectieuse de retard mental et de surdité congénitale contre lequel on essaie actuellement de développer un vaccin. On a testé trois doses de virus sauvages : 10 ufp, 100 ufp et 1 000 ufp. Chez les sujets séronégatifs, la dose de 10 ufp a été suffisante pour provoquer une infection. Chez les sujets séropositifs, ceux qui avaient donc eu une infection naturelle, seule la dose de 1 000 ufp a provoqué une infection. Enfin, les sujets vaccinés ont été protégés contre une dose de 10 ufp mais ont présenté une infection avec une dose de 100 ufp. Ces résultats témoignent bien de la puissance de l'immunité naturelle et de sa supériorité sur l'immunité vaccinale.

Quatrième leçon : il est relativement difficile d'immuniser les nourrissons et les personnes âgées

On sait que les anticorps maternels empêchent la vaccination. C'est la raison pour laquelle, par exemple, le vaccin contre la rougeole est administré à l'âge de 12 mois. De plus, même lorsqu'ils n'ont plus d'anticorps maternels, les nourrissons gardent un système immunitaire immature. Une étude incluant des enfants d'âges différents dont les anticorps maternels ont disparu montre qu'à l'âge de 12 mois ils présentent une excellente réponse à la vaccination rougeole ; en revanche à l'âge de 9 mois et plus encore à l'âge de 6 mois, la réponse à la vaccination est faible.
Le développement de vaccins polyosidiques conjugués, contre le pneumocoque ou le méningocoque, permet aujourd'hui de vacciner les nourrissons dès l'âge de deux mois. Le vaccin conjugué contre le méningocoque, par exemple, a de multiples avantages : il permet d'obtenir un titre d'anticorps plus élevé, il donne une mémoire immunitaire chez les jeunes enfants et il entraîne une réduction du portage du germe dans la gorge. Mais on sait aussi que l'efficacité de ce vaccin chez le nourrisson diminue fortement en l'absence de rappel.

Le méningocoque comporte 5 groupes pathogènes pour l'homme : A, B, C, W135 et Y. Un vaccin conjugué tétravalent A, C, W136 et Y est disponible aux États-Unis et est très utilisé chez les jeunes enfants et chez les étudiants. Il n'a pas été développé de vaccin conjugué pour le groupe B car les protéines de la capsule du méningocoque B ont une homologie avec une glycoprotéine du cerveau. D'autres stratégies ont donc été mises en œuvre pour obtenir un vaccin contre le méningocoque B. Dans un premier temps on a utilisé les protéines de la membrane externe des bactéries. L'efficacité d'un tel vaccin, évaluée dans une étude réalisée au Brésil, s'est révélée, là encore, très faible chez les nourrissons de moins de deux ans, partielle chez les enfants plus âgés et plus puissante chez les enfants d'âge scolaire. Ces expériences ont toutefois été une réussite car les vaccins ainsi conçus se sont révélés capables d'enrayer les épidémies d'infections à méningocoque. Ce type de vaccin contre le méningocoque B a été récemment utilisé en Nouvelle-Zélande, pays qui a connu une importante épidémie d'infections à méningocoque B. L'impact de la vaccination s'est très rapidement traduit par une forte diminution de ces infections. Dans l'avenir, une autre stratégie, la vaccinologie reverse, devrait permettre de développer un vaccin encore plus puissant contre le méningocoque B. Le principe de cette méthode repose sur le séquençage de la bactérie (600 gènes environ pour le groupe B) et la recherche des gènes pouvant produire des protéines de surface, qui ont la capacité d'induire la formation d'anticorps neutralisants. L'immunogénicité et la protection induite par ces protéines sont ensuite évaluées chez la souris. Le vaccin peut être réalisé à partir de l'une de ces protéines après s'être assuré qu'elle est conservée, c'est-à-dire qu'elle est présente dans toutes les souches bactériennes. Ce processus de fabrication est aujourd'hui bien avancé et l'on peut espérer disposer prochainement d'un nouveau vaccin contre le méningocoque de groupe B.

À l'autre extrémité de la vie, chez le sujet âgé, l'immunité est également moins puissante. Ainsi le vaccin grippal, par exemple, qui a une efficacité d'environ 80 % vis-à-vis des formes sévères de l'infection chez l'adulte jeune n'obtient que 48 % d'efficacité sur les hospitalisations et 50 % sur les décès chez les personnes âgées. Il n'est pas possible actuellement de parer à ce vieillissement du système immunitaire qui est lié à un épuisement des cellules B et T.

Cinquième leçon : les caractéristiques fonctionnelles des anticorps sont aussi importantes que leur quantité

L'exemple du vaccin polysaccharidique pneumococcique administré chez des sujets âgés l'illustre bien. Après vaccination, la réponse anticorps peut être évaluée de deux façons : par un test Elisa qui permet de détecter les anticorps fixés sur les antigènes et par un test fonctionnel qui étudie la capacité de phagocytose en mettant en contact le sang du sujet vacciné et la bactérie responsable de l'infection. Les sujets âgés de plus de 60 ans produisent des anticorps, mis en évidence par le test Elisa, mais relativement peu d'anticorps fonctionnels par rapport à des sujets jeunes. Ceci explique qu'un vaccin très efficace chez le sujet jeune ne le soit que modérément chez le sujet âgé.

Sixième leçon : l'immunité collective augmente avec l'efficacité des vaccins sur le terrain

En d'autres termes, l'efficacité d'une vaccination résulte de la protection conférée par le vaccin à chaque sujet vacciné mais également de l'immunité collective qui est liée à l'arrêt de la propagation de l'agent pathogène et qui permet aux sujets non vaccinés d'être eux aussi protégés. Ainsi, aux États-Unis, l'utilisation du vaccin contre le pneumocoque chez tous les enfants a abouti à une diminution spectaculaire des infections invasives ; elle a également eu pour conséquence une très forte réduction (55 %) des infections dues aux sérotypes contenus dans le vaccin chez les adultes vivant au contact des enfants vaccinés, tandis que l'incidence des infections liées aux autres sérotypes restait stable.

L'avenir

De nouvelles stratégies se développent actuellement et seront de plus en plus mises en œuvre dans l'avenir pour le développement de nouveaux vaccins : le réassortiment de segments de génomes de RNA, la génétique inverse, la recombinaison, la réplication, les plasmides ADN et d'autres stratégies encore. Mais le point le plus important pour le futur des vaccins est que la biologie moléculaire a ouvert la voie au développement de vaccins contre pratiquement toutes les maladies, à condition bien entendu que la pathogénie de la maladie soit connue.

La méthode de réassortiment a été utilisée pour la production d'un nouveau vaccin grippal vivant par voie nasale. Outre le fait que la voie nasale en facilite l'administration, ce vaccin a par ailleurs l'avantage de conférer une immunité plus large. Ainsi il induit une forte immunité non seulement lorsque la souche vaccinale et la souche circulante sont identiques mais également lorsqu'elles sont différentes, ce qui n'a jamais été constaté avec le vaccin inactivé. Le deuxième avantage de ce vaccin est de produire une immunité collective. Une étude menée dans deux villes du Texas a montré que la vaccination des enfants en milieu scolaire entraînait une réduction de l'absentéisme scolaire et des consultations médicales chez les enfants vaccinés mais également une diminution du nombre de congés maladie et de consultations médicales chez les adultes. Cette protection des adultes par le biais de la vaccination des enfants tient à une diminution du portage des souches grippales sous l'effet de la vaccination.

La recombinaison, autre stratégie nouvelle de développement des vaccins, a été mise en œuvre pour la fabrication d'un vaccin, encore expérimental, contre le virus *para-influenza* à l'origine d'infections respiratoires potentiellement graves chez le jeune enfant. Cette méthode a permis d'obtenir un vaccin recombinant contre les trois types de virus *para-influenza*. La recombinaison a également été utilisée pour la mise au point d'un vaccin contre le virus respiratoire syncytial. Ce vaccin a démontré son efficacité chez l'animal et est actuellement en cours de développement.

Enfin, un progrès majeur a marqué récemment le domaine de la vaccination : le développement d'un vaccin contre le papillomavirus humain (HPV) produit par la biologie moléculaire. L'infection à papillomavirus est une infection sexuellement transmissible qui affecte 50 % des femmes au cours de leur vie. Le plus souvent transitoires, ces infections peuvent, lorsqu'elles persistent, être à l'origine de dysplasies utérines et de cancers du col de l'utérus. Ce vaccin quadrivalent s'est révélé capable d'induire une protection de 100 %. Il devrait permettre d'éliminer la plupart des cancers utérins.

Les progrès récents dans les maladies héréditaires du métabolisme

Jean-Marie SAUDUBRAY

Consultant en maladies héréditaires du métabolisme,
Hôpital Necker-Enfants Malades, Paris, France

Les maladies héréditaires du métabolisme peuvent être classées en trois groupes. Le premier est celui des intoxications aiguës ou chroniques résultant d'erreurs innées du métabolisme intermédiaire ; la plupart des maladies de ce groupe sont traitables. Le deuxième groupe comporte les déficits énergétiques, également dus à des erreurs du métabolisme intermédiaire, mais dont seule une minorité est accessible à un traitement. Le troisième regroupe les anomalies de la synthèse ou du catabolisme des molécules complexes, parmi lesquelles plusieurs peuvent aujourd'hui être traitées efficacement.

Intoxications

Les erreurs innées du métabolisme responsables d'intoxication incluent les amino-acidopathies (phénylcétonurie, homocystinurie, tyrosinémie...), les aciduries organiques, les troubles du cycle de l'urée, les porphyries, les erreurs innées du métabolisme glucidique (galactosémie, intolérance héréditaire au fructose) et des métaux (maladies de Wilson, de Menkès, hémochromatose). Elles s'expriment souvent comme des urgences.

Certaines maladies par intoxication peuvent être traitées par les vitamines qui sont des cofacteurs des réactions enzymatiques. Si les connaissances sur les déficits du cycle de l'urée et les intolérances glucidiques ont peu évolué au cours des dernières années, des nouveautés sont à noter dans le domaine de la réponse à la vitamine B6. Des travaux récents ont révélé l'anomalie moléculaire impliquée dans l'épilepsie pyridoxino-dépendante. Cette maladie décrite il y a une cinquantaine d'années est due à des mutations du gène *ALDH7A1* qui code pour l'antiquitine [1]. Elle se caractérise par l'accumulation de P6C (acide piperideine-6-carboxylique), un composé très voisin du pyridoxal phosphate. Une autre maladie a été identifiée, associant un parkinsonisme et des convulsions, et ne répondant pas à la pyridoxine mais seulement au pyridoxal phosphate. Cette affection est la conséquence d'un défaut héréditaire de pyridox(am)ine-P oxydase qui empêche la transformation de la pyridoxine en son cofacteur, le pyridoxal phosphatase (métabolite actif de la vitamine B6).
Une aminoacidopathie, le déficit héréditaire de la synthèse de la sérine, s'est avérée particulièrement intéressante car elle représente le premier exemple de microcéphalie congénitale curable. L'administration de sérine à la mère durant la grossesse permet, en effet, de prévenir le développement de la microcéphalie [2, 3].
Une dernière nouveauté mérite d'être signalée dans le domaine des erreurs innées de la synthèse des acides aminés, à savoir l'identification du déficit en glutamine synthétase, qui se manifeste notamment par une atteinte du système nerveux central sévère [4, 5]. Cette découverte souligne pour la première fois le rôle neuroprotecteur important de la glutamine.

Déficits énergétiques

Les maladies héréditaires du métabolisme par carence énergétique peuvent être classées en deux catégories selon qu'elles affectent le processus énergétique cytoplasmique (glycogénose, déficit de la néoglucogenèse...) ou mitochondrial (acidémie lactique congénitale, déficits de la chaîne mitochondriale, déficits de l'oxydation des acides gras...). Ces pathologies ont fait et continuent de faire l'objet de nombreuses avancées parmi lesquelles la description de deux nouveaux groupes de maladies liées à un défaut de la synthèse de créatine cérébrale d'une part, et de la voie des pentoses phosphates d'autre part. Les déficits en créatine cérébrale entraînent des troubles neurologiques et représentent probablement une des causes fréquentes de retards mentaux liés à l'X. Ces retards mentaux sont parfois peu importants et se traduisent simplement par un retard de langage. Le bilan doit alors comporter une étude du pic cérébral de créatine par IRM spectroscopique. En ce qui concerne la voie des pentoses phosphates, les dernières données montrent un rôle majeur de cette voie dans le développement embryonnaire et représentent donc un champ de recherche fascinant.

Molécules complexes

Les maladies des molécules complexes rassemblent les maladies lysosomales, les maladies peroxysomales, les déficits de la synthèse endogène du cholestérol et les anomalies de glycolysation des protéines. C'est un domaine riche en avancées thérapeutiques et conceptuelles.
Depuis une dizaine d'années, des traitements substitutifs enzymatiques efficaces sont disponibles pour certaines de ces maladies comme celles de Gaucher, de Fabry, de Hunter, de Maroteaux-Lamy et de Pompe [6]. Par ailleurs, des travaux récents ont mis en évidence un phénomène d'empreinte parentale dans la maladie de Niemann-Pick [7]. Cette maladie, liée à un déficit en sphingomyélinase, se caractérise par une gravité extrêmement variable. On sait depuis peu que la sévérité du phénotype est conditionnée par l'allèle maternel.

En ce qui concerne les défauts de glycolysation des protéines, douze déficits de type I sont actuellement connus parmi lesquelles dix s'expriment par des troubles neurologiques et deux par une atteinte hépatique. Six maladies de type II, dont toutes sauf une impliquent le système nerveux central, ont été caractérisées. Les anomalies décrites portent sur la N-glycolysation mais aussi sur la O-glycolysation, ces dernières donnant des malformations cérébrales très graves et des myopathies, comme dans le syndrome de Walker-Warburg [8].

Enfin, les recherches sur la voie de la synthèse endogène du cholestérol montrent qu'il existe une maladie pour chaque étape et l'ensemble de ces maladies ont en commun de se manifester par des syndromes polymalformatifs.

Deux exemples illustratifs

Le déficit en glutamine synthétase

La glutamine est un acide aminé qui assure le transport de l'ammoniac. Elle est synthétisée essentiellement dans le muscle, mais également dans le foie. Deux cas de déficit en glutamine synthétase ont été rapportés en 2005 chez des nouveau-nés de parents turcs consanguins [4]. Le premier présentait un polyhydramnios avec des malformations cérébrales sévères (micromélie, kystes paraventriculaires, agyrie), insuffisance respiratoire, hypotonie, convulsions. Il est décédé au deuxième jour de vie. Le second avait une dysmorphie, des kystes subépendymaires, une microgyrie, des convulsions, une insuffisance respiratoire et une ascite, avec une issue fatale à quatre semaines. Dans les deux cas, le taux plasmatique de glutamine était quasiment nul (inférieur à 2 µmol/L).
Ces observations montrent, de façon inattendue, que la glutamine considérée uniquement comme un transporteur de l'ammoniac, a, en fait, un rôle très important dans la signalisation, l'apoptose et la prolifération cellulaires. Les effets dévastateurs du déficit profond en glutamine synthétase mettent également en lumière l'importance des besoins en glutamine pour le développement cérébral fœtal.

La voie des pentoses phosphates

La voie des pentoses phosphates a une double fonction : la production de ribose 5-phosphate nécessaire à la synthèse des acides nucléiques et la réduction de NADP (nicotinamide adénine dinucléotide phosphate) en NADPH, un cofacteur impliqué dans de nombreux processus de biosynthèse. Le glucose 6-phosphate déhydrogénase (G6PD) catalyse sa première étape.

En plus du déficit en G6PD, connu de longue date, deux maladies de cette voie viennent d'être décrites : le déficit en ribose-5-phosphate isomérase [9] et le déficit en transaldolase [10].
Des cas de déficit en transaldolase ont été rapportés au sein d'une famille turque hautement consanguine (parents cousins germains) ayant eu consécutivement quatre enfants atteints de la même affection [11]. Le premier est né à terme, avec un œdème généralisé, un placenta épais, une dysmorphie avec une implantation basse des cheveux, un hirsutisme et, surtout, un aspect de *cutis laxa*. D'autres signes étaient présents : une hépatomégalie avec insuffisance hépatocellulaire, une ané-

mie hémolytique avec leuconeutropénie et thrombocytopénie, une tubulopathie avec une néphrocalcinose et une condensation des os non confirmée ultérieurement. L'état neurologique de l'enfant était relativement conservé. Cet enfant est décédé à l'âge de cinq mois de son insuffisance hépatocellulaire après de nombreuses investigations qui n'ont pas permis de faire un diagnostic.

La deuxième grossesse, débutée deux ans après, a bénéficié d'une surveillance spécifique. Elle a été interrompue à vingt-six semaines en raison de multiples anomalies échographiques : retard de croissance, oligoamnios, placenta épais, dysmorphie, cardiomégalie, splénomégalie et ascite. Un message clinique peut être tiré de cette observation d'une forme particulière d'hydrops fœtal avec oligoamnios : le déficit en transaldolase doit être inscrit sur la liste des maladies à évoquer devant un tableau néonatal de ce type associé à une insuffisance hépatocellulaire avec hépatosplénomégalie, une dysmorphie et une anémie hémolytique récurrente. Un profil anormal des polyols doit être recherché car cette erreur innée du métabolisme se traduit par l'excrétion dans les urines d'érythritol, d'arabitol et de ribitol.

À l'occasion de travaux sur le rôle des polyols dans le développement fœtal, une équipe britannique a analysé des échantillons de sérum maternel et de liquide recueilli dans la cavité amniotique, la cavité cœlomique et l'espace intervillositaire juste avant des interruptions médicales de grossesse, à cinq-douze semaines [12]. Ce travail a montré qu'il existe une accumulation des polyols durant le premier trimestre de grossesse, à un moment du développement où la communication vasculaire du fœtus avec la mère est fermée. Dans cette période de développement, le fœtus vit donc en anoxie, mais il n'est pas en acidose. Sa seule source énergétique possible est le NADPH produit par la G6PD. C'est une voie peu rentable, mais élégante dans la mesure où elle produit de l'énergie sans acide lactique. Le même phénomène d'accumulation des polyols dans les liquides amniotiques et cœlomique a été observé dans la famille turque. Les polyols sont des molécules osmolytes qui contribuent probablement à l'accroissement du volume fœtal.

Ces données métaboliques originales doivent aussi être prises en compte dans la classification des anasarques, ouvrant ainsi la voie à un nouveau concept, aucune des classifications actuelles n'évoquant la notion d'osmolytes.

Références

1. Mills PB, Struys E, Jakobs C, *et al*. Mutations in antiquitin in individuals with pyridoxine-dependent seizures. *Nat Med* 2006 ; 12 : 307-9.
2. De Koning TJ, Klomp LW, van Oppen AC, *et al*. Prenatal and early postnatal treatment in 3-phosphoglycerate-dehydrogenase deficiency. *Lancet* 2004 ; 364 : 2221-2.
3. De Koning TJ. Treatment with amino acids in serine deficiency disorders. *J Inherit Metab Dis* 2006 ; 29 : 347-51.
4. Haberle J, Gorg B, Rutsch F, *et al*. Congenital glutamine deficiency with glutamine synthetase mutations. *N Engl J Med* 2005 ; 353 : 1926-33.

5. Haberle J, Gorg B, Toutain A, *et al*. Inborn error of amino acid synthesis : Human glutamine synthetase deficiency. *J Inherit Metab Dis* 2006 ; 29 : 352-8.
6. Desnick RJ. Enzyme replacement and enhancement therapies for lysosomal diseases. *J Inherit Metab Dis* 2004 ; 27 : 385-410.
7. Simonaro CM, Park JH, Eliyahu E, *et al*. Imprinting at the SMPD1 locus : implications for acid sphingomyelinase-deficient Niemann-Pick disease. *Am J Hum Genet* 2006 ; 78 : 865-70.
8. Beltran-Valero de Bernabé D, Currier S, Steinbrecher A, *et al*. Mutations in the O-mannosyltransferase gene POMT1 give rise to the severe neuronal migration disorder Walker-Warburg syndrome. *Am J Hum Genet* 2002 ; 71 : 1033-43.
9. Huck JH, Verhoeven NM, Struys EA, *et al*. Ribose-5-phosphate isomerase deficiency : new inborn error in the pentose phosphate pathway associated with a slowly progressive leukoencephalopathy. *Am J Hum Genet* 2004 ; 74 : 745-51.
10. Verhoeven NM, Huck JH, Roos B, *et al*. Transaldolase deficiency : liver cirrhosis associated with a new inborn error in the pentose phosphate pathway. *Am J Hum Genet* 2001 ; 68 : 1086-92.
11 Valayannopoulos V, Verhoeven NM, Mention K, *et al*. Transaldolase deficiency : a new cause of hydrops foetalis and neonatal multiorgan disease. *J Pediatr* 2006 ; 149 : 713-7.
12. Jauniaux E, Hempstock J, Teng C, Battaglia FC, Burton GJ. Polyol concentrations in the fluid compartments of the human conceptus during the first trimester of pregnancy : maintenance of redox potential in a low oxygen environment. *J Clin Endocrinol Metab* 2005 ; 90 : 1171-5.

Progrès en endocrinologie pédiatrique 2001-2006

Martin O. SAVAGE

*Department of Paediatric Endocrinology,
Barts and London School of Medicine, Londres, Royaume-Uni*

Au cours des cinq dernières années, l'endocrinologie pédiatrique a connu de très notables progrès qui ont modifié la pratique clinique. Lors d'une conférence donnée dans le cadre d'un colloque international Charles Nicolle, ont été présentés quelques-uns des progrès récemment enregistrés dans le domaine de la croissance et de son contrôle génétique.

Une croissance normale dépend de l'intégrité de l'axe GH-IGF-I (*growth hormone-insuline-like growth factor-I*) et résulte de l'effet conjugué de nombreux gènes. Ce contrôle polygénique de la croissance est bien illustré par la clinique, par les petites tailles idiopathiques par exemple, dans lesquelles on retrouve le plus souvent une petite taille parentale.

Insuffisance en GH et résistance à la GH

Les études de génétique moléculaire menées au cours des cinq dernières années ont permis de mettre en évidence certaines mutations à l'origine d'anomalies de la croissance. Rappelons qu'une mutation est une anomalie héritée dans la séquence de nucléotides de l'ADN à l'origine d'une anomalie de la structure de la protéine codée par ce gène. Il en résulte une perturbation d'un mécanisme endocrinien et par là un phénotype anormal. On a ainsi pu mettre en évidence une délétion de deux exons dans le gène de l'IGF-I à l'origine d'un dysfonctionnement de la protéine. Ceci se traduit par un taux élevé de GH, un taux indétectable d'IGF-I et cliniquement par un retard de croissance intra-utérin et une croissance postnatale anormale. Les travaux récents de génétique moléculaire ont également permis de caractériser des mutations à l'origine de déficits en GH et de déficit en IGF-I par résistance à la GH. On a pu ainsi identifier dans des cas d'insuffisance hypophysaire congénitale un déficit du gène PROP-1 à l'origine d'une absence de sécrétion de GH (ainsi que d'un déficit en ACTH).

La résistance à la GH est une autre cause d'anomalie de la croissance accessible aux investigations de génétique moléculaire depuis que l'on a identifié et cloné le gène du récepteur de la GH (GHR). Au cours des années 80-90, plusieurs mutations du gène du GHR ont été identifiées. La forme la plus sévère de résistance à la GH est le syndrome de Laron, maladie autosomique récessive liée à une insensibilité extrême à la GH en rapport avec des mutations au niveau du récepteur de la GH. Mais il apparaît aujourd'hui clairement que la population de patients résistants à la GH est en fait hétérogène. Une étude européenne portant sur 82 enfants présentant une résistance à la GH a ainsi montré qu'il existait au sein de cette entité diagnostique un spectre de sévérité allant du syndrome de Laron aux petites tailles idiopathiques. D'autres publications ont par la suite rapporté l'existence de mutations hétérozygotes chez certains enfants (dans une proportion estimée à 4 %) présentant une petite taille idiopathique. Un point important doit ici être précisé : chez les enfants de petite taille, l'étude du phénotype et la caractérisation des anomalies endocriniennes doivent toujours précéder la recherche éventuelle de mutations. L'expérience des années 80-90 a en effet montré que l'exploration de l'ADN réalisée en première intention ne donnait le plus souvent aucun résultat et qu'il était beaucoup plus productif d'identifier au préalable les anomalies endocriniennes.

La résistance à la GH peut également être liée chez certains patients à des anomalies situées plus bas dans la voie d'action de la GH, en aval du GHR, notamment au niveau de la molécule STAT5b. Le récepteur de la GH fait partie d'une famille de récepteurs incluant des récepteurs de cytokines et la molécule STAT5b joue un rôle dans la transmission intracellulaire de cytokines. Les patients présentant une mutation dans le gène de STAT5b ont à la fois une petite taille avec tous les signes biologiques de résistance à la GH (taux très bas d'IGFI, d'IGF-BP3 et d'ALS) et un déficit immunitaire lié à une perturbation de l'activité des cytokines.

Mutations dans le gène d'IGF-I et de son récepteur

En 1996 Woods et al. ont décrit le cas d'un enfant présentant une microcéphalie et une petite taille, avec sur le plan biologique un taux d'IGF-I indétectable et un taux d'IGF-BP3 normal (ce qui excluait une anomalie du récepteur de GH). Les explorations de biologie moléculaire ont permis de mettre en évidence chez cet enfant une anomalie du gène de IGF-I.

Une publication récente [1] a rapporté le cas d'un adulte présentant une petite taille (avec antécédent de retard de croissance intra-utérin), une surdité, une microcéphalie, un retard mental et une insulinorésistance. À la différence du patient décrit par Woods et al., ce patient hollandais avait un taux sérique d'IGF-I élevé. Les examens ont mis en évidence une mutation dans le gène d'IGF-I qui ne détruit pas complètement la protéine, mais la rend biologiquement inactive.

La présence d'un RCIU chez les patients présentant des mutations du gène d'IGF-I atteste du rôle fondamental que joue IGF-I dans la croissance fœtale.

Enfin, en 2003 un article paru dans le *New England Journal of Medicine* [2] a fait état de deux cas d'enfants présentant une mutation dans le gène du récepteur d'IGF-I.

Mutations dans le gène d'ALS

ALS (*acid labile subunit*) est une protéine qui lie IGF-I et BP-3. Dans la circulation, IGF-I se lie tout d'abord à BP-3 puis à ALS pour former un complexe ternaire qui constitue un réservoir d'IGF-I, biologiquement inactif. Le cas d'un patient présentant une mutation homozygote dans le gène de l'ALS a été publié en 2004 dans le *New England Journal of Medicine* [3]. Il s'agissait d'un homme de 20 ans avec une taille qui n'était que légèrement inférieure à la normale (1,69 m soit -0,5 DS) et chez lequel les examens biologiques ont montré un taux sanguin d'ALS indétectable et des taux également très bas d'IGF-I et de BP-3. Chez ce patient il existait une incapacité à former le complexe ternaire IGF-I-BP-3 et ALS. Cette coexistence d'un profil biochimique très anormal et d'une anomalie de croissance relativement peu importante tient à la persistance chez ce patient d'une production d'IGF-I paracrine, c'est-à-dire au niveau du cartilage de croissance, non affectée par la mutation.

En conclusion, les principales découvertes de ces cinq dernières années dans le domaine de la croissance peuvent être résumées en quelques points essentiels :

– La résistance ou l'insensibilité à la GH a un phénotype assez large qui va du syndrome de Laron aux petites tailles idiopathiques. La résistance à la GH est toutefois rarement en cause dans ces petites tailles idiopathiques.
– Parmi les défauts postrécepteurs, situés au niveau du processus de transduction du signal, les déficits en STAT5b peuvent être une cause de résistance à la GH qui est alors associée à des anomalies immunologiques.
– La croissance fœtale dépend de la production et de l'action normales d'IGF-I.
– Les mutations dans le gène de l'ALS sont à l'origine d'un défaut de croissance relativement peu marqué du fait du maintien d'une production paracrine d'IGF-I (au niveau du cartilage de croissance).

Enfin, il faut toujours garder à l'esprit que la caractérisation du phénotype et des anomalies endocriniennes du patient est un préalable indispensable avant toute exploration de génétique moléculaire.

Références

1. Walenkamp MJ, Karperien M, Pereira AM, et al. Homozygous and heterozygous expression of a novel insulin-like growth factor-I mutation. *J Clin Endocrinol Metab* 2005 ; 90 : 2855-64.
2. Abuzzahab MJ, Schneider A, Goddard A, et al. for the Intrauterine Growth Retardation (IUGR) Study Group. IGF-I receptor mutations resulting in intrauterine and postnatal growth retardation. *N Engl J Med* 2003 ; 349 : 2211-22.
3. Domene HM, Bengolea SV, Martinez AS, et al. Deficiency of the circulating insulin-like growth factor system associated with inactivation of the acid-labile subunit gene. *N Engl J Med* 2004 ; 350 : 570-7.

Nouveautés en pneumologie-allergologie pédiatrique

Pierre SCHEINMANN, *Rola* ABOU TAAM,
Jacques de BLIC, *Muriel Le* BOURGEOIS, *Chantal* KARILA

Hôpital Necker-Enfants Malades, Paris, France

L'analyse des progrès de ces 5 dernières années concernant l'asthme et les maladies allergiques constitue une haute priorité en raison de la prévalence des symptômes d'asthme, de rhinoconjonctivite allergique et d'eczéma chez l'enfant comme en témoignent les études ISAAC dont la dernière date de 2006 [1]. Pour la plupart des pays la prévalence de ces différentes affections augmente particulièrement chez les plus jeunes et plus particulièrement en ce qui concerne l'eczéma et la rhino-conjonctivite allergique. Les enquêtes épidémiologiques ne permettent pas de mettre en évidence un facteur unique à l'origine de cette augmentation. L'augmentation de prévalence, qui peut varier d'un pays à l'autre, d'une catégorie d'âge à une autre, doit faire envisager différents aspects du mode de vie, de l'alimentation, de la charge infectieuse [2], des conditions socioéconomiques, de l'environnement domestique et extérieur [3], de la variation climatique ainsi que de la prise de conscience de la maladie et de la prise en charge des symptômes.

L'augmentation de prévalence de l'asthme et des maladies allergiques concerne particulièrement les zones urbanisées ce qui correspond à notre mode vie occidentalisé. Ce phénomène d'urbanisation concerne également de manière croissante les pays en voie de développement [4].

L'idée relativement simpliste selon laquelle l'allergie crée l'asthme semble avoir vécu. La prévention primaire de l'allergie et de l'asthme est actuellement en situation d'échec. Dans ce même ordre d'idée la part de responsabilité des phénomènes allergiques IgE dépendants varie selon l'âge et l'affection en cause, de 30 % pour les sifflements répétés du nourrisson à 70-90 % pour l'asthme de l'enfant d'âge scolaire [5]. Chez l'enfant même si l'allergie ne peut plus être considérée comme le seul facteur pathogénique de l'asthme, l'asthme reste néanmoins une priorité pour l'allergologue. Cette priorité est d'autant plus élevée qu'il apparaît que les toutes premières années de la vie ont une importance fondamentale sur l'histoire dite naturelle des maladies allergiques et de l'asthme en particulier [6,7,8]. Il apparaît de plus probable que le pronostic de l'asthme à l'âge adulte se joue en très grande partie en période préscolaire [9].

Histoire naturelle de l'asthme et de l'allergie

Facteurs de persistance

Les enquêtes longitudinales montrent que c'est dans les 3 à 6 premières années de vie que s'installe au plan fonctionnel respiratoire un syndrome obstructif frappant les voies aériennes centrales et les voies aériennes périphériques [9]. L'enfant entre relativement tôt dans un couloir (phénomène du « *tracking* ») qui se poursuit chez le grand enfant [10,11] et jusqu'à l'âge adulte [12]. Les facteurs favorisant la chronicité et la persistance de l'asthme semblent bien être la sévérité et la précocité des symptômes, la sensibilisation aux allergènes perannuels, l'hyperréactivité bronchique, le sexe féminin, la puberté précoce, l'obésité et bien entendu le tabagisme [9].
L'irréversibilité des déficits fonctionnels respiratoires à l'âge adulte apparaît ainsi corrélée à l'importance du syndrome obstructif durant la première enfance [12].
Deux questions se posent donc avec acuité. Quelle est la physiopathologie de l'asthme persistant et particulièrement de l'asthme persistant sévère, voire difficile à traiter ? Les thérapeutiques anti-inflammatoires classiques (corticothérapie inhalée) peuvent-elles prévenir un processus paraissant peu ou pas réversible ?

Physiopathologie

Le remodelage bronchique

La physiopathologie de l'asthme et particulièrement de l'asthme sévère a fait l'objet de revues générales récentes [13, 14]. L'asthme sévère, qui concerne 5 à 10 % des enfants et des adultes asthmatiques, a pour caractéristiques d'être peu ou pas sensible aux corticoïdes inhalés même à forte dose, d'être à l'origine d'une morbidité voire d'une mortalité notables : c'est le phénotype d'asthme destiné à perdurer tout au long de la vie. Les acteurs anatomopathologiques de l'asthme concernent toute la paroi bronchique, aussi bien celle des bronches proximales que celle des bronches distales. Le remodelage bronchique a été particulièrement bien exploré par les auteurs européens qui ont étudié l'asthme de l'enfant [15, 16, 17]. Leurs travaux montrent bien la précocité des lésions, l'importance des phénomènes inflammatoires avec l'intervention non seulement des éosinophiles mais aussi des neutrophiles (en particulier chez le nourrisson et dans l'asthme difficile à traiter), la constance de l'épaississement de la membrane basale, lésions que l'on retrouve toutes dans l'asthme de l'adulte. Cependant il apparaît qu'outre l'altération de la fonction épithéliale et l'augmentation des réponses mésenchymateuses, un élément très important dans l'altération des fonctions respiratoires est représenté par l'hypertrophie et l'hyperplasie des muscles lisses et par l'angiogénèse excessive. Ces altérations de la paroi bronchique ont été parfaitement mises en évidence par Benayoun chez l'adulte asthmatique sévère avec syndrome obstructif [18]. Nos résultats préliminaires obtenus chez des enfants porteurs d'asthme sévère, âgés de 8 à 14 ans, montrent que l'hypertrophie et l'hyperplasie des muscles lisses bronchiques et le développement excessif de la vascularisation sont directement corrélés à l'importance du syndrome obstructif (données non publiées). Ces données nouvelles montrent donc que le remodelage bronchique, dans son aspect majeur de gravité, s'installe tôt dans la vie. Un élément péjoratif de l'histoire de l'asthme sévère est que ce type de remodelage est peu ou pas sensible à la corticothérapie inhalée. Il faut en effet noter que le processus de remodelage et les phénomènes inflammatoires semblent évoluer en parallèle ce qui ne les empêche pas de tisser des liens relativement étroits. Cependant le fait qu'une certaine inflammation ne puisse plus être considérée comme responsable du remodelage pose des problèmes d'avenir et des problèmes thérapeutiques.

La barrière épithéliale

L'intérêt attaché au développement excessif de la musculature lisse et des vaisseaux n'incite aucunement à négliger le rôle, probablement primordial, de l'épithélium bronchique dans la physiopathologie de l'asthme et l'entretien des processus de remodelage. Il apparaît même que le rôle de l'épithélium va s'étendre depuis les bronches jusqu'aux autres tissus impliqués dans la diathèse allergique : les muqueuses nasale et conjonctivale. Le déficit épithélial conduisant à une perte de son intégrité et à une augmentation de sa perméabilité facilite l'action nocive des divers irritants dont les virus et l'accès des allergènes, via les mastocytes, aux couches profondes des différents tissus [2,19].

Cette fragilité épithéliale aboutissant à une réparation défectueuse source de maladie chronique, conduit au plan pratique à tenter de réparer cet épithélium, et à accorder une place très importante à la protection des voies aériennes et de la peau contre les agressions environnementales. On voit que l'inflammation seule devient insuffisante à expliquer les origines de l'asthme chez l'enfant, que d'autres phénomènes mal expliqués interviennent, que l'environnement au sens large du terme a une importance croissante, et que les interactions gènes-environnement doivent être absolument prises en considération [3].

La fragilité et la perméabilité excessive des épithéliums démontrées également au niveau conjonctival sont peut-être liées à des altérations génétiquement transmises de certains constituants de l'épithélium. Tel est le cas de la peau : des anomalies congénitales de la filaggrine ont été démontrées chez les enfants porteurs d'eczéma et qui semblent obéir à l'hérédité récessive autosomique. Une partie des eczémas de l'enfant s'accompagne de mutations entraînant une perte de fonction de la filaggrine. La peau devient ainsi plus perméable, plus fragile. Le syndrome phénotypiquement délimité d'eczéma, d'allergie et d'asthme semble en partie trouver une explication génétique. Le déficit de filaggrine facilite l'acquisition de désordres allergiques touchant aussi bien les voies aériennes supérieures que les voies aériennes inférieures [20]. Le fait que les patients avec déficit en fillagrine et dermatite atopique soient également à risque accru d'asthme suggère la possibilité d'une sensibilisation allergénique par voie transdermique [21].

La barrière épithéliale et les allergies alimentaires

La réparation et le maintien d'intégrité de la barrière épidermique chez le nourrisson pourraient alors constituer un moyen de prévention des maladies allergiques des voies aériennes [22]. Lack *et al.* ont montré que parmi les facteurs associés au développement de l'allergie à l'arachide chez l'enfant, la présence d'un eczéma actif et évolutif combinée à l'application malencontreuse de thérapeutiques locales contenant de faibles doses d'arachide favorise l'allergie à l'arachide, c'est-à-dire un des plus grands problèmes d'allergie alimentaire auquel est confrontée notre société occidentale. L'hypothèse était donc que l'inflammation cutanée favorisait la sensibilisation à certains allergènes alimentaires, sensibilisation probablement favorisée par un terrain génétique particulier. Ce travail permettait également de souligner l'action probablement nocive des petites doses d'allergènes (sur terrain prédisposé) [23]. Cette intervention de l'allergie alimentaire dans certains aspects physiopathologiques de l'asthme sévère est d'autant plus importante à prendre en considération qu'il existe des liens entre sévérité de l'asthme et présence d'allergies alimentaires [24].

Populations lymphocytaires

Il est donc nécessaire de s'attacher à approfondir la physiopathologie de l'asthme sévère. Certains résultats récents méritent d'être soulignés :
Le rôle des lymphocytes Natural Killer CD4 + invariants a ainsi été mis récemment en exergue aussi bien chez l'animal que chez l'homme. Ces lymphocytes Natural Killer T invariants sont retrouvés chez l'enfant atteint d'asthme sévère. Leur proportion paraît plus faible que chez l'adulte, ce qui pourrait suggérer qu'elle augmente progressivement avec l'âge. Il est à noter que ce taux de lymphocyte T Natural Killer invariant n'est pas retrouvé dans d'autres pathologies telles la sarcoïdose, les dilatations des bronches, ni chez les contrôles. Il pourrait donc s'agir d'une sous-population lymphocytaire dont l'activité mériterait d'être bloquée [25, 26, 27].

Difficultés thérapeutiques

Histoire « naturelle »

Les plus récentes études longitudinales montrent que la corticothérapie inhalée même débutée très précocement ne modifie pas l'histoire naturelle de l'asthme du petit enfant [28]. Ce point souligne que des mécanismes biologiques différents sont à l'origine de la progression et de la symptomatologie de l'asthme. Les corticoïdes inhalés sont efficaces sur la symptomatologie, améliorent les fonctions respiratoires mais semblent s'avérer en pratique incapables de bloquer l'évolution naturelle de la maladie. Cette notion est très importante en pratique, car plus l'enfant est jeune, plus le diagnostic d'asthme au sens classique du terme est difficile à porter. Il existe donc un risque de traitement excessif des nourrissons siffleurs avec la possibilité soulevée par plusieurs auteurs que la corticothérapie puisse même inhiber le développement normal des voies aériennes qui survient pendant les derniers mois de la gestation et les premières années de la vie. Un traitement prolongé par corticoïdes inhalés ne peut donc être institué sans réflexion approfondie et éventuellement ne pas être entrepris avant qu'un phénotype clairement établi ne soit évident. Il est cet égard l'essai préliminaire d'immunothérapie de l'adulte avec un pollen (Amb a 1) conjugué à une séquence immunostimulante d'ADN (CpG) agoniste du TLR9 est très encourageant [41-44].

Le nourrisson et l'enfant d'âge préscolaire atteints d'asthme sévère méritent une attention toute particulière. Les objectifs sont d'éviter que le tout jeune asthmatique n'emprunte une voie nocive. Les cinq prochaines années permettront – peut-être – de déterminer quand et par quels procédés thérapeutiques le capital respiratoire du nourrisson asthmatique sévère pourra être réellement préservé.

Références

1. Asher MI, Montefort S, Bjorksten B, Lai CK, Strachan DP, Weiland SK, Williams H ; ISAAC Phase Three Study Group. Worldwide time trends in the prevalence of symptoms of asthma, allergic rhinoconjunctivitis, and eczema in childhood : ISAAC Phases One and Three repeat multicountry cross-sectional surveys. *Lancet* 2006 ; 368 : 733-43.
2. Holgate ST. Rhinoviruses in the pathogenesis of asthma : the bronchial epithelium as a major disease target. *J Allergy Clin Immunol* 2006 ; 118 : 587-90.
3. Vercelli D. Mechanisms of the hygiene hypothesis-molecular and otherwise. *Curr Opin Immunol* 2006 ; 18 : 733-7.
4. Mavale-Manuel S, Alexandre F, Duarte N, et al. Risk factors for asthma among children in Maputo (Mozambique). *Allergy* 2004 ; 59 : 388-93.
5. Scheinmann P. The course of allergy : what remains of the so-called natural history of allergy ? *Revue française d'allergologie et d'immunologie clinique* 2006 ; 46 : 402-7.
6. Guilbert TW, Morgan WJ, Zeiger RS, et al. Atopic characteristics of children with recurrent wheezing at high risk for the development of childhood asthma. *J Allergy Clin Immunol* 2004 ; 114 : 1282-7.
7. Illi S, von Mutius E, Lau S, et al. for the Multicentre Allergy Study (MAS) group. Perennial allergen sensitisation early in life and chronic asthma in children : a birth cohort study. *Lancet* 2006 ; 368 : 763-70.
8. Host A, Andrae S, Charkin S, et al. Allergy testing in children : why, who, when and how ? *Allergy* 2003 ; 58 : 559-69.
9. Sears MR, Greene JM, Willan AR, et al. A longitudinal, population-based, cohort study of childhood asthma followed to adulthood. *N Engl J Med* 2003 ; 349 : 1414-22.
10. Delacourt C, Benoist MR, Waernessyckle S, et al. Relationship between bronchial responsiveness and clinical evolution in infants who wheeze : a four-year prospective study. *Am J Respir Crit Care Med* 2001 ; 164 : 1382-6.
11. Delacourt C, Benoist MR, Waernessickle S, et al. Devenir des nourrissons asthmatiques : résultats de la cohorte des enfants malades à neuf ans. *Revue Française d'Allergologie et d'Immunologie Clinique* 2005 ; 45 : 530-2.
12. Limb SL, Brown KC, Wood RA, et al. Irreversible lung function deficits in young adults with a history of childhood asthma. *J Allergy Clin Immunol* 2005 ; 116 : 1213-9.
13. Boxall C, Holgate ST, Davies DE. The contribution of transforming growth factor-beta and epidermal growth factor signalling to airway remodelling in chronic asthma. *Eur Respir J* 2006 ; 27 : 208-29.
14. Holgate ST, Polosa R. The mechanisms, diagnosis, and management of severe asthma in adults. *Lancet* 2006 ; 368 : 780-93.
15. Barbato A, Turato G, Baraldo S, et al. Epithelial damage and angiogenesis in the airways of children with asthma. *Am J Respir Crit Care Med* 2006 ; 174 : 975-81.

16. Pascual RM, Peters SP. Airway remodeling contributes to the progressive loss of lung function in asthma : an overview. *J Allergy Clin Immunol* 2005 ; 116 : 477-86 ; quiz 487.
17. Chanez P, De Blic J, Delacourt C, et al. Characteristics of mild asthma : descriptive epidemiology and nature of bronchial inflammation. Position of the Mild Asthma Working Group. *Rev Mal Respir* 2006 ; 23: 17-28.
18. Benayoun L, Druilhe A, Dombret MC, et al. Airway structural alterations selectively associated with severe asthma. *Am J Respir Crit Care Med* 2003 ; 167 : 1360-8.
19. Lazaar AL, Panettieri RA Jr. Airway smooth muscle : a modulator of airway remodeling in asthma. *J Allergy Clin Immunol* 2005 ; 116 : 488-95 ; quiz 496.
20. Hudson TJ. Skin barrier function and allergic risk. *Nat Genet* 2006 ; 38 : 399-400.
21. Ying S, Meng Q, Corrigan CJ, Lee TH. Lack of filaggrin expression in the human bronchial mucosa. *J Allergy Clin Immunol* 2006 ; 118 : 1386-8.
22. Marenholz I, Nickel R, Ruschendorf F, et al. Filaggrin loss-of-function mutations predispose to phenotypes involved in the atopic march. *J Allergy Clin Immunol* 2006 ; 118 : 866-71.
23. Lack G, Fox D, Northstone K, Golding J. Avon Longitudinal Study of Parents and Children Study Team. Factors associated with the development of peanut allergy in childhood. *N Engl J Med* 2003 ; 348 : 977-85.
24. Wang J, Visness CM, Sampson HA. Food allergen sensitization in inner-city children with asthma. *J Allergy Clin Immunol* 2005 ; 115 : 1076-80.
25. Kay AB. Natural killer T cells and asthma. *N Engl J Med* 2006 ; 354 : 1186-8.
26. Pham-Thi N, de Blic J, Le Bourgeois M, et al. Enhanced frequency of immunoregulatory invariant natural killer T cells in the airways of children with asthma. *J Allergy Clin Immunol* 2006 ; 117 : 217-8.
27. Pham-Thi N, de Blic J, Leite-de-Moraes MC. Invariant natural killer T cells in bronchial asthma. *N Engl J Med* 2006 ; 354 : 2613-6.
28. Guilbert TW, Morgan WJ, Zeiger RS, et al. Long-term inhaled corticosteroids in preschool children at high risk for asthma. *N Engl J Med* 2006 ; 354 : 1985-97.
29. Simpson A, Soderstrom L, Ahlstedt S, et al. IgE antibody quantification and the probability of wheeze in preschool children. *J Allergy Clin Immunol* 2005 ; 116 : 744-9.
30. Walker S, Monteil M, Phelan K, Lasserson TJ, Walters EH. Anti-IgE for chronic asthma in adults and children. *Cochrane Database Syst Rev* 2006 ; 19 : CD003559.
31. Bousquet J, Cabrera P, Berkman N, et al. The effect of treatment with omalizumab, an anti-IgE antibody, on asthma exacerbations and emergency medical visits in patients with severe persistent asthma. *Allergy* 2005 ; 60 : 302-8.
32. Humbert M, Beasley R, Ayres J, et al. Benefits of omalizumab as add-on therapy in patients with severe persistent asthma who are inadequately controlled despite best available therapy (GINA 2002 step 4 treatment) : INNOVATE. *Allergy* 2005 ; 60 : 309-16.
33. Berry MA, Hargadon B, Shelley M, et al. Evidence of a role of tumor necrosis factor alpha in refractory asthma. *N Engl J Med* 2006 ; 354 : 697-708.
34. Erzurum SC. Inhibition of tumor necrosis factor α for refractory asthma. *N Engl J Med* 2006 ; 354 : 754-8.
35. Ballow M. Biologic immune modifiers : Trials and tribulations-are we there yet ? *J Allergy Clin Immunol* 2006 ; 118 : 1209-15.
36. O'Byrne PM. Cytokines or their antagonists for the treatment of asthma. *Chest* 2006 ; 130 : 244-50.
37. Moller C, Dreborg S, Ferdousi HA, et al. Pollen immunotherapy reduces the development of asthma in children with seasonal rhinoconjunctivitis (the PAT-study). *J Allergy Clin Immunol* 2002 ; 109 : 251-6.
38. Norman PS. Immunotherapy : 1999-2004. *J Allergy Clin Immunol* 2004 ; 113 : 1013-23.
39. Scheinmann P. Immunotherapy in young children. In : Lockey RF. *Allergens and Allergen Immunotherapy.* New York : Marcel Dekker Inc, 2004 ; 567-83.
40. Eng PA, Borer-Reinhold M, Heijnen IA, Gnehm HP. Twelve-year follow-up after discontinuation of preseasonal grass pollen immunotherapy in childhood. *Allergy* 2006 ; 61 : 198-201.

41. Simons FE, Shikishima Y, Van Nest G, *et al.* Selective immune redirection in humans with ragweed allergy by injecting Amb a 1 linked to immunostimulatory DNA. *J Allergy Clin Immunol* 2004 ; 113 : 1144-51.

42. von Baehr V, Hermes A, von Baehr R, *et al.* Allergoid-specific T-cell reaction as a measure of the immunological response to specific immunotherapy (SIT) with a Th1-adjuvanted allergy vaccine. *J Investig Allergol Clin Immunol* 2005 ; 15 : 234-41.

43. Crameri R, Rhyner C. Novel vaccines and adjuvants for allergen-specific immunotherapy. *Curr Opin Immunol* 2006 ; 18 : 761-8.

44. Creticos PS, Schroeder JT, Hamilton RG, *et al.* Immune Tolerance Network Group. Immunotherapy with a ragweed-toll-like receptor 9 agonist vaccine for allergic rhinitis. *N Engl J Med* 2006 ; 355 : 1445-55.

Les progrès récents en nutrition

Yvan VANDENPLAS*

*Clinique pédiatrique, Academisch Ziekenhuis Kinderen,
Vrije Universiteit Brussel, Bruxelles, Belgique*

Les problèmes nutritionnels dans le monde varient selon le lieu. Quantitatifs dans les pays en développement, ils sont essentiellement de nature qualitative dans les régions développées. Cette revue traite des champs concernés par les avancées récentes en nutrition à l'exclusion de l'obésité, du syndrome métabolique, des antioxydants et des radicaux libres.

Les infections gastro-intestinales

Les infections gastro-intestinales aiguës et chroniques ont un impact majeur sur la morbidité et la mortalité infantiles dans le monde. Certains germes, principalement le rotavirus, *Escherichia coli* entéropathogène, les salmonelles, *Giardia lamblia* et les cryptosporidies, entraînent des lésions intestinales persistantes, dont la sévérité est augmentée par une nutrition et une réalimentation inadéquates. De nombreuses études méthodologiquement solides ont évalué l'efficacité de l'adjonction, aux solu-

---

* Rédaction : Catherine Faber, d'après la communication d'Yvan Vandenplas au Colloque Charles Nicolle de Rouen.

tés de réhydratation orale (SRO), de substances de type glycine, alanine, glutamine, oligosaccharides, ou de l'utilisation comparative de riz et de glucose. Aucune d'entre elles ne permet de conclure à la supériorité de ces solutés « enrichis » sur les SRO « classiques ». À l'heure actuelle, une seule voie semble intéressante, celle de l'adjonction de zinc au SRO qui permet de raccourcir la durée de la diarrhée et de diminuer la mortalité, y compris chez les enfants infectés par le VIH [1]. Ces bénéfices du zinc s'expliquent par ses effets antioxydants et sur la croissance [2].

Dans les gastroentérites aiguës, la mise en œuvre d'une réalimentation rapide a permis de diminuer l'incidence du syndrome postentéritique. Les hydrates de carbone complexes, les probiotiques et prébiotiques, ainsi que la L-glutamine, les nucléotides, le colostrum bovin sont en cours d'évaluation.

La maladie cœliaque

L'augmentation de la prévalence de la maladie cœliaque (MC) notée dans le monde s'explique, en grande partie, par l'amélioration du dépistage sérologique des sujets ne présentant pas de troubles gastro-intestinaux. Cette évolution se caractérise toutefois par l'émergence de différences régionales. On note également une grande variabilité – encore inexpliquée – de l'âge d'apparition des symptômes, des manifestations extradigestives et auto-immunes, de la séropositivité et de la sévérité des lésions histologiques.

Le constat d'une incidence plus élevée de la MC chez les femmes ayant accouché prématurément que dans la population générale soulève le problème de l'évolution de la grossesse lorsque le diagnostic est méconnu et du statut nutritionnel du nouveau-né.

Sur le plan histologique, quatre types de MC ont été décrits, le troisième ayant été récemment sous-catégorisé en 3a, 3b et 3c (classification de Marsh). Pour la NASPGHAN (*North American Society for Pediatric Gastroenterology, Hepatology and Nutrition*), l'association de lésions de types 1 et 2, d'anticorps positifs et d'une réponse sérologique et clinique positive au régime sans gluten signe le diagnostic de MC [3]. Des données supplémentaires sont nécessaires sur le niveau d'observance des patients asymptomatiques, le risque réel de complications dans les lésions de type 1, le seuil de sensibilité au gluten et la signification clinique de la séropositivité en l'absence d'entéropathie. Il en est de même pour le rôle de l'allaitement maternel prolongé, le moment de l'introduction du gluten et les doses contenues dans les aliments, en particulier chez les sujets à haut risque génétique.

Parmi les pistes de recherche thérapeutique figurent la supplémentation en peptidase, la modulation de la perméabilité intestinale, un blé transgénique sans peptides antigéniques et le blocage de l'immunité innée et acquise. Enfin, des efforts doivent être menés en vue de définir précisément les modalités du régime sans gluten, de simplifier l'étiquetage des produits alimentaires, d'améliorer la prise en charge sociale des patients et leur identification précoce.

Les allergies alimentaires

Ces dernières décennies ont été marquées par une augmentation du nombre d'enfants sensibilisés à plusieurs trophallergènes, même en cas d'allaitement maternel prolongé, avec des manifestations allergiques précoces. Outre la symptomatologie digestive, bien connue, les allergies alimentaires peuvent se manifester par des symptômes extradigestifs qui, chez l'enfant, sont souvent prédominants.

Différentes données émergent de la littérature récente :
– sur le plan histologique, le constat, sur des biopsies duodénales, d'une réduction de l'expression de TGF-bêta 1 +, à la fois au niveau de l'épithélium et au niveau de la lamina propria, ainsi qu'au niveau des cellules mononuclées et de l'épithélium [4] ;
– l'absence de preuves définitives de l'efficacité préventive des interventions diététiques durant la grossesse [5] ;
– chez les nourrissons à haut risque, l'intérêt en cas d'impossibilité d'allaitement au sein prolongé des hydrolysats de protéines pour réduire la prévalence des allergies alimentaires et des allergies aux protéines de lait de vache, et ce sans différence significative entre les hydrolysats partiels et poussés [6].

Les gastroentéropathies et œsophagites à éosinophiles

Rares en Europe, les entéropathies éosinophiliques ont une physiopathologie et une approche thérapeutique variables selon leur type : gastroentéropathie et œsophagite à éosinophiles sont des entités spécifiques différentes. Le rôle primaire des trophallergènes et des aéroallergènes dans leur pathogénie reste à établir.

En raison d'un aspect macroscopique de la muqueuse souvent normal à l'endoscopie, leur diagnostic nécessite l'analyse de multiples échantillons biopsiques. Ces affections se manifestent cliniquement par divers symptômes comme des vomissements, une dysphagie, des douleurs abdominales, une diarrhée, une anémie ferriprive, des troubles de la croissance, une ascite séreuse…

Dans certains cas, des tentatives d'exclusion d'allergènes alimentaires et aériens sont réalisées. La corticothérapie générale ou locale peut donner de bons résultats, en particulier dans les œsophagites. De nombreux autres traitements ont été testés, sans résultats probants [7], comme le cromoglycate, le montelukast, le ketotifène, le mycophénolate mofétil, des antagonistes de CCR3 (chemokine receptor-3).

La maladie de Crohn

La maladie de Crohn est une maladie multifactorielle impliquant des facteurs immunitaires, génétiques et environnementaux. Plusieurs arguments confortent l'importance de la flore intestinale dans son développement, à savoir l'absence de maladie dans des conditions de flore stérile, l'association avec des mutations du gène *NOD2* qui code une molécule intracellulaire importante dans la réponse inflammatoire aux peptidoglycanes bactériens, et la production d'interferon-gamma induite chez les patients par des extraits de leur propre flore commensale.

Les effets bénéfiques potentiels des probiotiques ont été remis en cause par une récente étude randomisée contre placebo dans laquelle *Lactobacillus rhamnosus* souche GG (associé au traitement standard) n'a pas entraîné d'augmentation de la durée de la période sans rechutes [8]. De nombreuses études d'intervention diététique ont été réalisées, sans résultats significatifs. D'après le Comité de nutrition de la Société française de pédiatrie, les solutions polymériques de nutrition entérale et les solutions élémentaires ou semi-élémentaires ont la même efficacité. L'alimentation entérale nocturne prolongée présente un grand intérêt chez les enfants ayant un retard staturo-pondéral ou pubertaire et dans les formes corticorésistantes ou corticodépendantes [9]. Des progrès ont été faits dans la compréhension des mécanismes d'action de l'alimentation entérale. Les auteurs d'une revue Cochrane récente soulignent le besoin urgent de réaliser de larges études multicentriques sur les différents traitements de la maladie de Crohn chez l'enfant et de standardiser les modalités de mesure de la croissance [10].

Les nutriments

Si la supplémentation en *glutamine* semble associée à une diminution de la morbidité et de la mortalité infectieuses, l'alimentation entérale enrichie en ce nutriment n'améliore pas la tolérance alimentaire ou l'évolution à court terme des bébés de petit poids de naissance. En outre, l'analyse des résultats des études randomisées de bonne qualité méthodologique montre que cette supplémentation n'a aucun bénéfice clinique significatif chez les prématurés [11].

Les *nucléotides* ont récemment fait l'objet de plusieurs études expérimentales et cliniques. Chez l'animal, les régimes avec nucléotides ont des effets bénéfiques sur la croissance et la maturation gastro-intestinales, la réparation des lésions intestinales et l'immunité cellulaire et humorale, et, par ailleurs, entraînent une augmentation des taux de survie après injection d'agents pathogènes. Chez les nourrissons, ce type de régime est associé à une plus faible incidence de diarrhée et à une augmentation des anticorps après administration du vaccin anti-*hæmophilus influenzæ* B. Enfin, l'ajout de nucléotides à l'alimentation des bébés avec retard de croissance intra-utérin sévère a des effets bénéfiques sur la microflore intestinale, l'incidence des diarrhées et la fonction immunitaire [12]. Il faut toutefois souligner que les laits enrichis en nucléotides n'ont pas les mêmes bénéfices que le lait maternel.

Des apports adéquats en *lipides* sont importants en termes de couverture des besoins caloriques, mais aussi du fait de leurs effets immunomodulateurs. Une étude animale suggère ainsi que les triglycérides à chaînes moyennes ont des propriétés antivirales et antibactériennes [13]. Une revue Cochrane récente ne retrouve pas de différence significative de la croissance à court terme, de l'intolérance digestive et de l'incidence des entérocolites nécrosantes chez les prématurés nourris avec une formule lactée contenant des acides gras à chaînes moyennes ou longues [14]. Comme pour les nucléotides, le rapport coût/bénéfice de l'enrichissement d'acides gras polyinsaturés à longues chaînes dans les laits infantiles reste discuté [15].

Des études cliniques ont mis en évidence les effets des laits enrichis en *oligosaccharides* sur la flore digestive des nouveau-nés prématurés et à terme [16]. Cette supplémentation ne modifie pas les taux de cholestérol et de triglycérides évalués à l'âge de six mois. L'adjonction de prébiotiques au lait ou aux céréales infantiles diminue la consistance des selles des nourrissons [17] et module l'immunité cellulaire. Le Comité nutrition de l'ESPGHAN (*European Society for Paediatric Gastroenterology Hepatology and Nutrition*) estime que s'il n'existe pas de preuves de l'intérêt des prébiotiques et des oligosaccharides, ils n'entraînent pas d'effets secondaires [18].

En ce qui concerne les *probiotiques*, une étude contrôlée contre placebo a montré que *Bifidobacterium bifidum* et *Streptococcus thermophilus* préviennent les diarrhées nosocomiales chez les nourrissons hospitalisés au long cours [19]. Les effets des probiotiques sont spécifiques à une souche. Les résultats observés avec une souche ne peuvent donc pas être extrapolés à d'autres. Les probiotiques illustrent bien l'évolution vers la nutrithérapie et les problèmes de législation des suppléments alimentaires qui en découlent.

Références

1. INCLEN Childnet Zinc Effectiveness for Diarrhea (IC-ZED) Group. *JPGN* 2006 ; 42 : 300-5.
2. Baqui AH, Ahmed T. Diarrhoea and malnutrition in children. *BMJ* 2006 ; 332.
3. Hill ID, Dirks MH, Liptak GS, et al. North American Society for Pediatric Gastroenterology, Hepatology and Nutrition. Guideline for the Diagnosis and Treatment of Celiac Disease in Children : Recommendations of the North American Society for Pediatric Gastroenterology, Hepatology and Nutrition. *J Pediatr Gastroenterol Nutr* 2005 ; 40 : 1-19.
4. Perez-Machado MA, Ashwood P, Thomson MA et al. Reduced transforming growth factor-Beta1 producing T cells in the duodenal mucosa of children with food allergy. *Eur J Immunol* 2003 ; 33 : 2307-15.
5. Salvatore S, Keymolen K, Hauser B, Vandenplas Y. Intervention during pregnancy and allergic disease in the offspring. *Pediatr Allergy Immunol* 2005 ; 16 : 558-66.
6. Osborn DA, Sinn J. Formulas containing hydrolysed protein for prevention of allergy and food intolerance in infants. *Cochrane Database Syst Rev* 2003 ; 4 : CD003664.
7. Rothenberg ME. Eosinophilic gastrointestinal disorders. *J Allergy Clin Immunol* 2004 ; 113 : 11-28.
8. Bousvaros A, Guandalini S, Baldassano RN, et al. A randomized, double-blind trial of Lactobacillus GG versus placebo in addition to standard maintenance therapy for children with Crohn's disease. *Inflamm Bowel Dis* 2005 ; 11 : 833-9.
9. Beattie RM. Enteral nutrition as primary therapy in childhood Crohn's disease : control of intestinal inflammation and anabolic response. *J Parenter Enteral Nutr* 2005 ; 29 (4 Suppl) : S151-5.
10. Newby EA, Sawczenko A, Thomas AG, Wilson D. Interventions for growth failure in childhood Crohn's disease. *Cochrane Database Syst Rev* 2005 ; 3 : CD003873.
11. Tubman TR, Thompson SW, McGuire W. Glutamine supplementation to prevent morbidity and mortality in preterm infants. *Cochrane Database Syst Rev* 2005 Jan 25 ; 1 : CD001457.
12. Yu VY. The role of dietary nucleotides in neonatal and infant nutrition. *J Paediatr Child Health* 2002 ; 38 : 543-9.
13. Kono H, Fujii H, Asakawa M, et al. Medium-chain triglycerides enhance secretory IgA expression in rat intestine after administration of endotoxin. *Am J Physiol Gastrointest Liver Physiol* 2004 ; 286 : G1081-9.
14. Klenoff-Brumberg HL, Genen LH. High versus low medium chain triglyceride content of formula for promoting short term growth of preterm infants. *Cochrane Database Syst Rev* 2003 ; 1 : CD002777.
15. Field CJ, Clandinin MT, Van Aerde JE Polyunsaturated fatty acids and T-cell function : implications for the neonate. *Lipids* 2001 ; 36 : 1025-32.
16. Bakker-Zierikzee AM, Alles MS, Knol J, et al. Effects of infant formula containing a mixture of galacto- and fructo-oligosaccharides or viable Bifidobacterium animalis on the intestinal microflora during the first 4 months of life. *Br J Nutr* 2005 ; 94 : 783-90.
17. Moore N, Chao C, Yang LP, et al. Effects of fructo-oligosaccharide-supplemented infant cereal : a double-blind, randomized trial. *Br J Nutr* 2003 ; 90 : 581-7.
18. Agostoni C, Axelsson I, Goulet O, et al. ESPGHAN Committee on Nutrition. Prebiotic oligosaccharides in dietetic products for infants : a commentary by the ESPGHAN Committee on Nutrition. *J Pediatr Gastroenterol Nutr* 2004 ; 39 : 465-73.

19. Saavedra JM, Bauman NA, Oung I, Perman JA, *et al.* Feeding of Bifidobacterium bifidum and Streptococcus thermophilus to infants in hospital for prevention of diarrhoea and shedding of rotavirus. *Lancet* 1994 ; 344 : 1046-9.

Recent Advances in
General Paediatrics

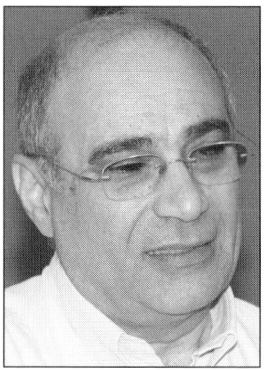

Recent Advances in Paediatric Gastroenterology

Samy CADRANEL

Department of Gastroenterology, Queen Fabiola Children's Hospital, Free University of Brussels, Brussels, Belgium

Introduction

Paediatric gastroenterology has been recognized as a true specialty in its own right since the early seventies. Until then paediatricians involved in diseases of the GI tract dealt mainly with diarrhoeal diseases and nutrition, especially malnutrition. Intensive research on coeliac disease gave an initial input to this new specialty which still lacked specific characteristics and tools. The discovery during those years of two "new" infectious agents of the GI tract, namely *campylobacter* and rotavirus, and the important role they played, was a further step towards recognition of this specialty in paediatrics. During approximately the same period modern fiberoptic endoscopy was developed as a clinical tool in adult patients and, shortly afterwards also in children.

Endoscopy has benefited from technical improvements and new instruments as well as devices that enable better diagnostic and therapeutic procedures. Some 20 years ago it enabled another important discovery in the field of peptic diseases. The dogma that the stomach, because of its acidic contents, remains almost "germ-free" was shattered by the discovery of *Helicobacter pylori*, and its role in chronic peptic diseases and as a co-carcinogen. Although the mechanisms of transmission of *Helicobacter pylori*, present in more than half of the human population world wide are still poorly understood. However, it is widely accepted that the infection is mainly acquired during infancy.

Due to the recent "destitution" of cisapride, many changes have occurred in the management of another important intensively studied topic, gastro-oesophageal reflux (GER).

In the industrialized regions of the world, food allergies and eosinophilic oesophagitis together with inflammatory bowel diseases beginning in childhood seem to be increasing whereas accidental caustic oesophagitis still remains frequent in the developing world. New treatment strategies are emerging.

The purpose of this article was to briefly review the main advances or changes that have occurred during the past five years in the field of paediatric gastroenterology.

Gastro-oesophageal reflux

GER is an extremely common and usually self-limiting condition in infants and considered as physiological in normal infants. It requires no specific treatment in uncomplicated cases. However, regurgitation is poorly accepted by the family and many anti-regurgitation (AR) formulas, based on adjunction of thickening agents, have been commercialized. Rice cereal is used predominantly in the United States while locust bean gum, at a concentration of 0.45 g/100 ml, is the most frequent thickening agent used in Europe. The efficacy of this type of AR formula was reported in a randomized trial [1]. However, based on the frequency of the symptoms evaluated by the mothers, a less concentrated formula containing only 0.35 g/100 ml was found to be more effective than the regular thicker formula.

Gastro-oesophageal reflux disease (GERD) has been intensively studied during the past five years whether in improving the diagnostic methods, investigating the role of GER in extra-digestive symptoms or modifying the treatment options. Most published studies that link GERD to respiratory diseases have been limited by their small size, selection bias, lack of controls, narrow focus on a single respiratory problem, and the confounding effects of including patients with neurological disease or congenital oesophageal anomalies. To avoid these deficiencies a major case-control study on the association between GERD and respiratory disease was performed [2] using Texas Children's Hospital's administrative database. This major, intensive, epidemiological study has approached the issues regarding the association between GERD and respiratory disease better than any similar study to date. It has raised an important question regarding a negative association of GERD with otitis media. In a comment to this article [3], it was stressed that, if the authors' institution diagnoses approximately 500 children a year with GERD, of whom at least 13% have respiratory disorders, it should not take long to do a prospective, placebo-controlled, double-blind therapeutic trial, using modern exhaustive pharmacotherapy for GERD. Although this type of study could have delayed GERD therapy for children assigned to placebo, it did provide the basic data required to justify antireflux therapy in children with respiratory diseases.

For more than 20 years paediatricians have used prokinetics as the first step to treat GER and GERD. Despite millions of doses given throughout the world, cisapride has been questioned regarding its efficacy and safety. Reports of possibly serious adverse events, e.g. an increased QTc interval, cardiac arrhythmias, and death, associated with the use of cisapride and due to reports of fatal cardiac arrhythmias or sudden death, from July 2000, cisapride has been restricted to a limited access programme supervised by a paediatric gastroenterologist in the US and in Europe, to patients treated within a clinical trial or safety study or registry programme [4].

In a meta-analysis of randomized controlled trials of cisapride using a random-effects model of ten trials involving 415 children [5] there was no evidence of a significant reduction in vomiting severity with cisapride as measured by a clinical score. Twenty-four-hour oesophageal pH monitoring data showed the mean reflux index was significantly lower in the children treated with cisapride compared with controls. With cisapride treatment, there was also no reduction in the mean number of reflux episodes lasting longer than 5 min or in the number of children with oesophagitis at final follow-up compared with baseline. There was no significant difference in reported side-effects or adverse events. Finally no clinically important benefits of cisapride in children with GER have been demonstrated. Nor was there any evidence of adverse or harmful events.

In the absence of easily available and efficient prokinetics, alternative strategies are being developed addressing acid suppression [6]. Using the acid-inhibitory agents (histamine-2 receptor antagonists, proton pump inhibitors) are the most widely used. Numerous clinical studies performed in adults, and several studies involving children, have demonstrated that the proton pump inhibitors are more effective than the histamine-2 receptor antagonists in the relief of GERD symptoms and healing of erosive oesophagitis. Studies performed with omeprazole and lansoprazole in children have shown pharmacokinetic parameters that closely resemble those observed in adults. In over a decade of use in adults, the proton pump inhibitor class of agents has been found to have a good safety profile and in numerous drug-drug interaction studies performed with these two proton pump inhibitors, relatively few clinically significant interactions have been observed. Although some studies involving children have also shown these agents to be well tolerated, the example of the mismanagement of the "cisapride story" should induce caution when using such potent drugs for a prolonged period of time [7]. In a very recent report [8] the risk of acute gastroenteritis and community-acquired pneumonia is reported to have increased in children treated with gastric acidity inhibitors. In addition, this effect seems to be sustained even after the end of therapy as a result of many factors, including direct inhibitory effect of GA inhibitors on leukocyte functions and qualitative and quantitative gastrointestinal microflora modification. With the advent of PPIs, H2-receptor antagonists anti-secretory drugs tend to be less used. However, in a large recent study [9], the safety and efficacy of nizatidine seemed very promising. Gastro-oesophageal reflux disease is difficult to control with medical therapy in neurologically impaired children. The gamma-aminobutyric acid type B receptor agonist baclofen was recently reported to reduce reflux in adult patients with GERD by reducing the incidence of transient lower oesophageal sphincter relaxations. Baclofen (0.7 mg/kg/day) was administered orally or via nasogastric tube in three divided doses 30 minutes before meals for 7 days in eight neurologically impaired children with GERD with good results [10] reducing the frequency of emesis and the total number of acid refluxes.

Bile reflux has been postulated to be an important factor contributing to gastro-oesophageal reflux disease in adults. In a study involving 65 children [11] using ambulatory 24-hour oesophageal pH and bilirubin monitoring both bile and acid reflux increase stepwise with the severity of oesophagitis. The ability of bile acids to cause damage depends on both their conjugation status and pH [12]. Conjugated bile acids when pH < 4 can cause additional damage to oesophageal mucosa compared to refluxate at equivalent pH without bile acids present. However, with deconjugated bile acids at pH < 4 there is no additional damage as the deconjugated bile acids are precipitated out of solution. In a less acidic environment, deconjugated bile acids can cause oesophageal damage.

Out-patient 24-hour oesophageal pH-metry detects only acid GER and cannot answer the question of the possible harmful effect of non-acid GER. Its role as the gold standard method could be replaced by a new device (MII) combining pH monitoring and impedance measurement [13] which allows to characterize the proportion of acid and non-acid oesophageal reflux events in young infants with suspected GER. MII detects more reflux events than pH monitoring alone. Combined pH-MII oesophageal monitoring identifies more reflux events and improves clinical correlation with symptoms. The proportion of non-acid reflux to acid reflux events in infants is more similar to adults than previously reported [14]. This technique might prove helpful in elucidating the mechanisms involved in GERD with respiratory instead of digestive symptoms. A lower nasopharyngeal pH in children with chronic respiratory disease has also been recently reported [15] and could become a marker to select patients who should be included into a 24h oesophageal pH-metry although the lower nasopharyngeal pH could be due either to GER or to an inflammatory condition of the mucous system.

Childhood GERD might be a risk factor for GERD in adolescents and young adults [16] as overall 24 (30%) adult patients in a cohort of 80 identified as having GERD as children were still were currently taking either H2RA or PPI, and 19 patients had undergone fundoplication. This raises the possibility that GERD may have a genetic basis. The suspicion that GERD might have a familial component is not new [17]. The first reports of familial hiatal hernia were published nearly forty years ago. In the subsequent decades, two dozen publications have identified familial clustering of hiatal hernia (HH), Barrett's oesophagus (BE), oesophageal adenocarcinoma, and GERD. A specific locus associated with pediatric GERD has been identified on chromosome 13 and some evidence exists for a specific locus for pediatric GERD at 13q14.

Eosinophilic oesophagitis (EE)

The diagnostic hallmark of this "new" entity, known since 1982, is the presence of > 20 eosinophils/high power field within the oesophageal epithelium or deeper tissue levels. Symptoms are similar to those of GER but pH monitoring is usually normal and there is a poor response to anti-reflux therapy. There is a male predominance and main age of presentation is 10 years [18]. The frequent allergic antecedents and the good response to anti-allergic therapy lead to presume an allergic aetiology [19]. Is EE prevalence increasing or is it more frequently recognized in children? We should consider this disease in patients with long-standing symptoms presumed to be caused by atypical GER with bad response to anti-reflux therapy. A normal appearance of oesophageal mucosa at endoscopy should not prevent the clinician from obtaining biopsies for histopathological studies [20]. Although the beneficial effects of steroids have been well documented most of patients have very intermittent symptoms and the use of long-term oral steroids is not justified [21]. A range of presenting symptoms in children with EE have been improved by ingested fluticasone propionate [22]. More recently montelukast, a leukotriene receptor antagonist (LTRA) which actively and selectively blocks the leukotriene D4

(LTD4) receptor has also been used with promising results. Because LTD4 is both produced by and a chemotactic factor for eosinophils, this may provide the rationale for treating a patient with EE [23].

Caustic oesophagitis

Ingestion of caustic compounds (strong alkaline or acid substances) by children is almost always accidental and leads to severe lesions of the oesophagus. Whereas the frequency of these accidents is decreasing in the industrialized regions of the world, mainly due to prevention by legal measures regarding packaging and labelling, it remains a true concern due to the squalor or poor living conditions of the developing world.

What is the best attitude in order to prevent the inevitable consequence of narrow oesophageal strictures? The major clinical question after a suspected caustic ingestion is to correctly evaluate the degree of injury and to predict which patients are at risk for development of complications. Currently, endoscopy is the only widely accepted method of assessing the depth and extent of injury [24]. There have been multiple grading scales devised to assess the extent of oesophageal or gastric injury after a caustic ingestion. In the majority of cases, grade 0 indicates no injury, grade 1 is injury limited to the mucosa characterized by oedema or erythema, and grade 2 indicates penetration to the submucosa with ulceration or whitish membranes. Grade 2 injury is usually divided into superficial, non-circumferential ulceration and deeper more circumferential lesions. Grade 3 injury is associated with transmural involvement with deep injury, necrotic mucosa, or frank perforation of the oesophagus or stomach. Patients with grade 0 or 1 burns can be fed as tolerated and discharged home after the endoscopic procedure. Patients with grade 2 injury are usually fasted until the extent of the injury becomes clear. If signs of perforation do not develop, the patients may be fed but should be observed for the possible development of oesophageal stricture. Patients with grade 3 burns usually (but not always) require a prolonged period of no intake by mouth and intravenous nutrition. Antibiotics are indicated when confronted with perforation and are often used in conjunction with steroids in patients with severe mucosal injury.

The role of steroids remains controversial, but they are used by many clinicians in patients with severe non-perforating mucosal damage. Recently it has been confirmed [25] that the use of the "regular" 2 mg/kg dose of prednisolone has no beneficial effect. On the contrary, experimental studies on rabbits have shown that high doses of dexa-methazone could partially prevent oesophageal strictures and this trend was also observed in 1996 in children. The results of the multicentre trial conducted by the French speaking group of paediatric gastroenterology, hepatology, and nutrition (GFHGNP) with very large doses of methyl-prednisolone, initiated as soon as possible after the ingestion confirm these results [26, 27].

Endoscopic dilatations become necessary when oesophageal strictures develop. Other endoscopic techniques have been proposed in order to reduce the number of dilatations such as Poliflex stents [28] or an indwelling balloon [29]. These procedures require adequate equipment and extreme caution to avoid complications such as ulcerative oesophagitis [30] or perforations by the stent [31]. A new concept has recently emerged advocating the use of mitomycin to stabilise and reduce the number of dilatations required [32].

Helicobacter pylori gastritis

The 2005 Nobel Prize for Medicine was awarded to Barry Marshall and Robin Warren for their discovery of the role of *Helicobacter pylori* (HP) as the bacteria that infects more than half of the world's human stomachs. During these two decades its role as the major factor responsible for chronic peptic diseases has been unquestionably proven as well as its role as a co-carcinogen in the progression towards MALT and gastric carcinoma. Only a few years after this important discovery HP was also found in children. Although the transmission of the infection is poorly understood it is widely accepted that contamination occurs in early life, especially in developing regions of the world, hence influencing the research in this field by paediatric gastroenterologists. It is well documented that in high prevalence regions almost all children and infants are contaminated very early. HP infections in mothers and siblings and birth in high-prevalence countries stand out as strong markers of infection risk together with poor social conditions and living in squalor [33]. At what age does it occur in the developed countries? In an important recent study [34] 327 healthy index children between 24 and 48 months of age were enrolled over 15 months. At baseline, the HP infection status of each index child and their older siblings and parents was assessed by using the carbon 13-urea breath test. All non-infected index children were then followed up with an annual carbon 13-urea breath test for 4 years to determine whether they became infected with HP and, if so, the age at first infection. The rate of infection per 100 person-years of follow-up was highest in the 2-3-year age group (5.05 per 100 person-years of follow-up) and declined progressively as children aged. Only 1 child became infected after 5 years of age. The question whether breast-exclusive feeding may protect against HP infection is an important issue [35]. The HP seropositivity of a large cohort of 407 individuals born in 1947 was investigated and related to the duration of exclusive breastfeeding after adjusting for measures of socioeconomic status and adverse housing conditions at birth. An increased duration of exclusive breastfeeding in infancy may have a long-term protective effect against chronic HP infection and hence the risk of gastric carcinoma. These data may prove important for promoting breast-feeding in the developing world. The re-infection rate is more common in children than in adults. Adolescents become re-infected, whereas acquisition of primary *H pylori* infection occurs predominantly in early childhood. Close contact with young children, especially siblings, younger than 5 years could be a more important risk factor than the age of the patient at the time of treatment for the high rate of re-infection in childhood [36]. Besides *Helicobacter pylori* other *Helicobacter spp* can co-exist in the stomach of individuals. Using PCR, *H pylori* was detected in 75 (83.3%), *H felis* in 23 (25.6%), and co-infection in 21 (23.3%) of 90 South African volunteers. *H felis* was randomly distributed among adults and children but clustered within families, suggesting intrafamilial transmission. Analysis of histopathology scores revealed no differences in atrophy, activity, and *helicobacter* density between *H felis*-positive and *H felis*-negative volunteers [37].

In the early period of the HP era many papers were published associating HP gastritis with recurrent abdominal pain in children. Although a consensus has been reached whereby no such specific symptoms can be identified, unexpected differential associations with strain specific infections may indicate a so far overlooked complex relationship [38]. A follow-up of a cohort of 347 children in day care centres showed a significant and non-transient effect of infection caused by HP on height and weight [39]. Another very large study addressing the same question [40] involved 2932 participants aged 40-49 years: HP infected men were 0.7 cm shorter than uninfected men (NS) whereas infected women were 1.4 shorter than uninfected ones. Although *H pylori* infection is associated with reduced adult height in women, this may be due to residual confounding factors. Less controversial is the influence of HP gastritis on iron deficiency which has been documented in papers originating from countries with very different climates such as Finland [41], Turkey [42] and Alaska [43].

When dealing with children, non-invasive diagnostic methods are always preferred to invasive ones. The detection of HP antigens in stools has been known in recent years but not fully accepted, especially in younger children [44]. However, better results obtained with monoclonal antibody-based enzyme immunoassay, make this test a promising technique for epidemiological studies.

First-line treatment of HP gastritis based on Bismuth salts regimens, which proved to be an inexpensive and rather efficacious solution in the 80s and 90s has been progressively replaced by the more expensive scheme based on the combination of

2 antibiotics and one PPI. The same type of regimen is commonly used for the treatment of HP infection in children and in adults but with lower eradication rates [45]. The increasingly growing frequency of resistant HP strains is probably responsible for the somewhat disappointing results [46]. Other therapies are under scrutiny such as the combined use of *Clostridium butyricum* which reduces the changes in the intestinal flora and decreases the incidence of gastrointestinal side effects [47]. Pro- and prebiotics have also been tried such as *Lactobacillus LB* or *Saccharomyces Boulardii* with inulin. The latter could be helpful in reducing the bacterial load [48]. Other therapeutic approaches have addressed the bactericidal and anti-adhesive properties of different plants against HP. Among the plants that killed *H pylori (in vitro)*, turmeric was the most efficient, followed by cumin, ginger, chilli, borage, black caraway, oregano and liquorice. Moreover, extracts of turmeric, borage and parsley were able to inhibit the adhesion of *H pylori* strains to stomach sections [49]. Another approach involves the development of specific phenolic profiles with optimisation of different ratios of extract mixtures from oregano and cranberry [50].

Although HP infection is acquired in early childhood the clinical and histological picture differs in children and adults. IFN-gamma secretion in the stomach of *H pylori*-infected patients is lower in children than in adults. This could protect children from development of severe gastro-duodenal diseases such as ulcer diseases. In addition, infected patients are characterised by a dysregulation of mucosal cytokine secretion at distance from the infection site [51]. A predominant Th1 profile has been demonstrated in *H. pylori*-infected mucosa from adults while the cytokine response appeared to be smaller in HP-infected children than in adults without a clear Th1 dominance [52]. These results therefore suggest a different mucosal immunopathology in children where the gastric immune response could be down-regulated in children with HP infection. Atrophy of the gastric mucosa, accepted as a first step towards metaplasia and malignancy, is very rare in children. However, Japanese authors [53] report a prevalence of 10.7% of grade 2 or 3 atrophy and 4.6% metaplasia in the antrum of 196 children aged 1-16 years. The same trend seems to be observed in Algerian children (personal communication).

Endoscopy

The role of endoscopy in gastroenterology is paramount and it has become an indispensable tool also in paediatric gastroenterology. The technology has greatly progressed from the times of rigid endoscopy with sophisticated lenses to fiberoptics which allowed flexibility and miniaturized processors in the video-endoscopes, which greatly improve the quality of the images and facilitates therapeutic procedures by multidisciplinary specialized teams. Paediatric GI endoscopy has benefited from the mandatory miniaturization for its use in small children and infants and also from the progresses in anaesthesia and sedation [54]. Upper GI tract and colon, as well as the distal segment of the ileum can be explored leaving only the small bowel relatively out of reach even with long enteroscopes, difficult in practice to use in paediatrics [55]. New instruments, such as the double balloon endoscopy [56] are being developed which can explore the small bowel but also obtain biopsies and even perform therapeutic procedures.

Undoubtedly, the wireless capsule endoscopy represents the newest and more popular device, widely discussed in the medical literature but also in the media, popular newspapers and magazines. The concept of swallowing a capsule slightly more voluminous than a drug tablet instead of having to undergo invasive endoscopy is certainly appealing but still has limited indications. The procedure is expensive, time-consuming and does not allow an on-line procedure guided by the endoscopist nor to obtain biopsies or perform direct therapeutic interventions. The size of the capsule partially limits its indications in young children; fortunately small bowel bleeding, the main indication in adults, is not frequent in childhood. A few papers have been published in paediatrics as case reports [57] or as larger series review [58] where new indications such as Crohn's and coeliac diseases are included. Technical improvements are being planned which will probably render easier the cumbersome reading of the recordings. The reduction in price would probably increase the number of procedures with better defined new indications.

Together with miniaturisation of the instruments the progress made in anaesthesiology have also played an important role in the development of paediatric GI endoscopy. There are still controversies in the literature regarding general anaesthesia, light or deep sedation with a combination of drugs such as ketamine [59] or propofol [60] or even no sedation at all in "motivated children" [61]. However, the same authors confess that the 80% of those non-sedated "motivated children" would prefer general anaesthesia if a second endoscopy is required. In our experience any combination with ketamine is difficult to manage and propofol needs the presence of an anaesthesiologist. Almost unknown in the US, equimolar mix of oxygen and nitrogen monoxide is easy, well tolerated and frequently used in France and Belgium.

Percutaneous endoscopic gastrostomy (PEG) is probably the only procedure of GI endoscopy initiated in children before its use in adult patients. Complications are not rare, mainly because PEG is used in fragile and difficult patients. In a series of 110 children [62] the overall rate of late-onset complications was 44% (48 complications observed in 29 patients – 26%). 75% of the complications appeared during the first 2 years after PEG insertion. Nine different types of complication have been identified. To properly answer the question of the relationship between PEG and

GER, future studies should address the following points [63], which are still a source of confusion or debate. Can we rely on pH-metry to study GER in such patients, since the use of continuous enteral feeding can lead to the presence of buffered gastric material that makes the diagnosis of acid GER very difficult? Has the location of gastrostomy (antral versus fundus) any effect on the occurrence or worsening of GER? What is the exact influence of the type of enteral nutrition (continuous versus bolus)? Is PEG by itself the main factor influencing the outcome of GER, or do other factors (enteral nutrition modalities or nutritional rehabilitation) also play a role in this relationship?

Inflammatory bowel disease

Once considered rare in paediatric practice, chronic inflammatory bowel disease (IBD) is now being recognized with increasing frequency in children of all ages. In IBD, growth failure may be the only clinical presentation and it is imperative to perform a detailed history and physical examination to search for other systemic and gastrointestinal manifestations of the disease. IBD can have a significant impact on linear growth, weight gain, and bone mineralization, and can cause delays in the onset of puberty [64]. Twenty-five per cent of inflammatory bowel disease occur in childhood. Growth and nutrition are key issues in the management with the aim of treatment being to induce and then maintain disease remission with minimal side-effects. Only 25% of Crohn's disease (CD) present with the classic triad of abdominal pain, weight loss, and diarrhoea. Most children with ulcerative colitis (UC) have blood in the stool at presentation. Inflammatory markers are usually although not invariably raised at presentation, particularly in CD. Full investigation includes upper gastro-intestinal endoscopy and ileocolonoscopy [65].

For a number of years CD seemed to be present only in the developed areas of the world and especially in Caucasians. This pattern seems less and less likely to be the rule in Western Europe and North America where many children from immigrant parents are now living. This trend has been studied in the UK. In Bangladeshis in East London, the incidence of IBD has increased whereas that of abdominal tuberculosis has fallen over the past decade. Clinicians in the Western world need to be aware of the changing incidences of IBD and abdominal tuberculosis in South Asians [66]. The same experience applies to other migrant populations not only from North Africa in France and Belgium and from Turkey in Germany but also from Central Africa.

Continuous spikes and waves during slow sleep (CSWS)

Dysgraphia may be specifically involved in relation to CSWS [39].

Absence epilepsy

Early-onset absences may be associated with paroxysmal dystonia (kinesigenic, exercise-induced or tonic upgaze) that occurs later than the absences and persist for a longer period [40].

Frontal lobe epilepsy

New specific tasks may reveal distinct cognitive troubles, and the capacity to resist the interference of a distracter is selectively affected [41]. Following surgery, patients improve in terms of attention and in short and long-term memory [42].

Rasmussen encephalitis (RE)

By 4 to 6 months following the first symptoms, MRI shows high signal on T2-weighted images in the cortex and white matter, cortical atrophy usually involving the frontoinsular region, with mild or severe enlargement of the lateral ventricle and moderate atrophy of the head of the caudate nucleus [43, 44].
Clinical *variants* include bilateral cases, particularly in the young age [45] and cases with progressive facial atrophy of the Parry-Romberg syndrome [46].
GluR3 antibodies affect 4% [47] to 64% [48] of patients with pharmacoresistant focal epilepsy compared to 7% and 82% in RE. Preliminary data with immunosuppressive compounds seem encouraging although they comprise a serious risk of severe infectious complications [49, 50].

Previously undescribed patterns

Although *hyperekplexia* is considered to be distinct from epilepsy, rare families exhibit a combination of both with a dramatic outcome [51].
The combination of *spinal muscular atrophy and progressive myoclonic epilepsy* has been reported in sporadic patients [52] and families [53].

Status epilepticus (SE)

Young age at onset and symptomatic aetiology independently favour SE [54]. Mortality is low [55] and outcome similar to that of patients without SE [56].

Devastating epilepsy of school age child (DESC) begins between 4 and 10 years with status epilepticus triggered by fever and lasting several weeks. Patients may die without inflammation in the brain [57]. Following SE and without any silent period, survivors remain with intractable perisylvian epilepsy, severe amnesia and speech troubles [58]. Memory troubles are correlated with bilateral hippocampal damage [59]. Although some ability to learn remains, memory troubles have major impact on everyday life [60].

During SE, the increased demand for energy leads to *complete depletion of glycogen reserves* [61].
The combination of SE with hypoglycaemia generates brain lesions, including HH syndrome [62].

Aetiology

Inborn errors of metabolism

Mitochondriopathies. Infantile spasms (IS) are a predominant manifestation of epilepsy, they may occur alone or in association with partial seizures [63]. Bilateral putaminal necrosis may be associated with infantile spasms and the T8993G NARP mutation [64]. Blood lactate may be normal, particularly when IS are the only seizure type [65].

Polymerase (DNA directed), gamma (POLG) mutations are responsible for mitochondrial DNA depletion that causes Alpers syndrome, often without respiratory chain abnormalities in skeletal muscle [66].

Menkes disease has a recognizable pattern with focal seizures starting as a status epilepticus in the first year of life, followed by West syndrome one or 2 years later [67].

GLUT1 deficiency syndrome (GDS). EEG is slow on fasting. Focal anomalies affect infancy and generalized spike-wave children. Seizure types include absences, myoclonus, partial, and astatic fits [68]. Atypical absences respond to ketogenic diet [69].

Pyridoxine-dependant seizures (PDS) and pyridoxal phosphate dependency. PDS result from a mutation in the antiquitine gene that codes for the enzyme catabolizing alpha-aminoadipic semialdehyde (α-AASA) which chelates pyridoxine [70]. Detection of α-AASA in urine, not altered by pyridoxine administration, provides a simple means to establish biochemical diagnosis whereas ALDH7A1 gene analysis permits prenatal diagnosis.

Pyridoxal phosphate dependency is due to a mutation in the PNPO gene encoding pyridox(am)ine 5'-phosphate oxidase and produces a similar pattern [71].

Inherited impairment of mitochondrial glutamate transport [72] also causes neonatal myoclonic encephalopathy (NME). The common denominator for the 4 conditions (glycine encephalopathy, pyridoxine dependency, pyridoxal phosphate dependency and glutamate transporter deficiency) is the increased glutamate/GABA ratio in the synaptic clefts. Inhibition of glutamate transporters experimentally produces the same pattern [73].

Folate and B12 deficiency. Cerebral folate deficiency (CFD) produces developmental delay, psychomotor regression, seizures, and autistic features reversible with folinic acid administration. CSF level of 5-methyltetrahydrofolate is low [74].

Chromosomopathies, monogenic encephalopathies and related disorders

The characteristics of seizures in *4p- Wolf-Hirschhorn syndrome* are an onset within the first 2.5 years with unilateral seizures [75]. The frequency of both seizures and status epilepticus decreases gradually after 5 years of age [76].

Ring chromosome 20 (RC20). One case has been reported with onset in the neonatal period and posterior predominance of abnormalities [77].

In *CDKL5/STK9* mutations, epilepsy starts before the age of 3 months, with myoclonic seizures and tonic spasms [78-80].

Mutations in the *ARX* gene have been reported in combination with either epilepsy consisting of myoclonic seizures or infantile spasms (hypsarrhythmia being a rare feature) [81].

Malformations

Cortical dysplasia. Intrapartum complications could lead to misdiagnosis [82]. Pharmacoresistant partial seizures contrast with easily treatable spasms [83]. In patients with additional hippocampal sclerosis (dual pathology) febrile seizures are significantly more frequent than reported in patients without dual pathology. Both the dysplastic tissue and the sclerotic hippocampus are epileptogenic [84].

Hemimegalencephaly. Hemimegalencephaly is sporadic, 30% have underlying neurocutaneous syndromes [85]. Contralateral hemimicrencephalia could explain cognitive troubles and seizure relapse following surgery [86].

Periventricular nodular heterotopia. Ictal EEG and SEEG recordings suggest that seizures are generated by abnormal anatomic circuitries including the heterotopic nodules and adjacent cortical areas [87], and may be combined with overlying polymicrogyria [88].

Hypothalamic hamartoma (HH). Isolated HH causes more severe seizures and neurological dysfunction and more early-stage puberty than when it is part of Pallister-Hall syndrome (PHS) where infantile spasms often occure late [89]. Transcallosal resection of HH is effective for pharmacoresistant epilepsy, with 76% of patients becoming seizure-free or having > 90% seizure reduction [90, 91].

Bilateral perisylvian polymicrogyria combined with clubfoot suggests prenatal ischemia [92]. Generalized polymicrogyria with perisylvian predominance is not familial [93] whereas bilateral frontoparietal polymicrogyria (BFPP) is autosomal recessive and maps to chromosome 16q12-21 [94].

Tumours

Angiocentric neuroepithelial tumour is congenital, benign but distinct from dysplastic neuroepithelial tumour: angiocentric polarity, positive gliofibrillary acidic protein (GFAP) and fusiform and bipolar astrocytic cells are arranged around blood vessels in the cortical grey matter and white matter with a stalk like extension to the ventricle [95].

Febrile seizures (FS) and later epilepsy

The type of epilepsy syndrome following FS is determined by the characteristics of the FS: they are significantly longer and more focal when followed by temporal lobe epilepsy, whereas brief generalized seizures are followed by generalized epilepsy [96].

MRI within 48 hours following a unilateral prolonged FS may show hippocampal oedema that has disappeared 4 months later, leaving hippocampal asymmetry with smaller hippocampus contralateral to the side of the convulsion but without the other signs of sclerosis [97].

Age at onset in mesial temporal lobe epilepsy with a history of FS is determined by the age at the first FS. The age at FS is earlier in the adolescent than in the childhood epilepsy onset group [98]. Neocortical development abnormalities predominate in case of onset before 5 years [99]. *Cortical dysplasia* is a common finding in intractable temporal lobe epilepsy (21/33), even in cases with a history of febrile convulsions (11/15), CNS infection (2/3) or familial history of epilepsy (5/6) [100]. Hippocampectomy is less likely to be effective in children than in adults [101] because it fails to remove the affected neocortex responsible for the early onset of the epilepsy.

Leukaemia may be complicated by hippocampal sclerosis, probably as a result of prolonged seizures generated by *antileukemic treatment* [102], particularly intrathecal methotrexate [103].

The relationship between *hippocampal dysgenesis* and seizures remains unclear. Hippocampal asymmetry without sclerosis on MRI exhibits a positive family history of epilepsy, low incidence of febrile seizures and benign prognosis, suggesting that this entity is distinct from hippocampal sclerosis [104]. Although reported in adults, hippocampal sclerosis without epilepsy [105] is never incidental in paediatrics [106].

Brain maturation and epilepsy

Brain maturation facilitates epilepsy and epilepsy delays brain maturation. Therefore, both contribute to pharmacoresistance.

Spike foci predominate more often the left hemisphere from the age of 5 years, whereas earlier, right foci predominate [107]. This is consistent with the later maturation of the left hemisphere [108]. Status epilepticus in a patient with focal dysplasia damaged the contralateral hemisphere because it is the most excitable at this age [109].

Brain maturation largely contributes to epileptogenesis:
– Early in life GABA neurotransmission is mildly excitatory, the only excitatory neurotransmission since NMDA is under strict control, due to glutamate transporters. Increased NMDA transmission generates neonatal epilepsy with myoclonus and suppression-bursts.
– Synaptic excess involves both excitatory and inhibitory transmissions in infancy and childhood and results in the spike and slow wave pattern of BECTS and of many epileptic encephalopathies, *i.e.* CSWS and LGS. The lack of slow waves in the neonatal period (suppression-burst pattern) results from the lack of GABA inhibition.
– The synaptic excess involves different areas at different ages: the motor area at term permitting myoclonic activity, the parieto-occipital areas in infancy, generating visual agnosia in WS, and the frontal lobes in childhood, a characteristic of LGS.
– Spike asynchrony in hypsarrhythmia results from the lack of myelin (required for interhemispheric synchronization) before 18 months of age.
– Long distance connections appear progressively:
• Between the spinal cord and motor strip: somatotopy is generated by jerks produced by the spinal cord neurones: this could explain that:
 – since dysplastic neurones do not generate normal contacts, the latter are organized out of the dysplastic cortex, reducing the risk for motor defect following surgery;
 – progressive disappearance of neurones in case of endogenous toxicity would revert motricity to primordial pathways with jerks, a characteristic of progressive myoclonic encephalopathy.
• Between the neocortex and the hippocampus which is an amplifier producing episodic memory by the echo it produces in the neocortex, from the middle of the first decade.

Thus:
– the hippocampus damaged in infancy by prolonged focal convulsions may only produce very delayed epilepsy, in adolescence;
– premature development of hippocampal-neocortical pathways could cause the hippocampus to produce an echo in a still hyperexcitable neocortex, thus very severe status epilepticus as described under the heading "DESC" [110].

In severe epilepsy seizures semiology remains unchanged over decades, even on relapse [111]. Myelination is delayed in patients with severe early onset temporal lobe epilepsy [112]. GABAergic neurones in hippocampi removed from adult epileptic brain have reverted to the immature excitatory stage, contributing to pharmacoresistance [113]. Therefore, brain maturation is delayed in the structures involved in the generation of severe epilepsy.

Treatment

Drug treatment (AEDT)

Lamotrigine may induce seizure aggravation with negative myoclonus in idiopathic rolandic epilepsy [114]. The comparison of *buccal midazolam* to *rectal diazepam* produced variable results, from midazolam superiority [115] to equality [116, 117]. Benzodiazepines may remove the spikes in CSWS syndrome without improving the clinical condition [118].
The effect of Vigabatrin in infantile spasms was established comparing low to high doses [119], and no difference with the effect of steroids could be identified [120]. The risk for visual field constriction seems to be lower than for adults with the shortest duration of 15 months [121]. AEDT in epileptic encephalopathy may be antiepileptogenic, not only antiepileptic, particularly in infantile spasms, provided it is administered within the first 2 months of the disease [122].

Ketogenic diet (KD)

For stabilized conditions, initiating KD *without fasting* may be the best option. Patients lose significantly less weight, and have fewer and less severe episodes of hypoglycemia, acidosis and dehydration, but there is no difference in the incidence of vomiting [123].

Surgery

The likelihood of curing seizures in *hypothalamic hamartoma* seems to be higher when lesions are approached from above sessile rather than from below [124, 125] whereas approaches from below adequately expose pedunculated hamartomas.
Blood loss and duration of hospitalization are lower but incidence of seizure relapse higher with lateral disconnection [126]. Vertical disconnection could prevent seizure relapse while reducing blood loss and duration of hospitalization [127]

Prognostic and social aspects

Fever may cause remission of intractable epilepsy, particularly in WS and related conditions [128].

Most patients who relapse after treatment withdrawal regain seizure control [129]. In non surgical patients, approximately 1% relapse uncontrollably [130].

References

1. Korff C, Nordli DR, Jr. Do generalized tonic-clonic seizures in infancy exist? *Neurology* 2005; 65: 1750-3.
2. Nakazawa C, Fujimoto S, Watanabe M, *et al*. Eating epilepsy characterized by periodic spasms. *Neuropediatrics* 2002; 33: 294-7.
3. Pachatz C, Fusco L, Vigevano F. Epileptic spasms and partial seizures as a single ictal event. *Epilepsia* 2003; 44: 693-700.
4. Franzon RC, Montenegro MA, Guimaraes CA, *et al*. Clinical, electroencephalographic, and behavioral features of temporal lobe epilepsy in childhood. *J Child Neurol* 2004; 19: 418-23.
5. Ray A, Kotagal P. Temporal lobe epilepsy in children: overview of clinical semiology. *Epileptic Disord* 2005; 7: 299-307.
6. Fogarasi A, Janszky J, Tuxhorn I. Autonomic symptoms during childhood partial epileptic seizures. *Epilepsia* 2006; 47: 584-8.
7. Wyder-Westh C, Lienert C, Pihan H, Steinlin M. An unusual cause of stridor in childhood due to focal epileptic seizures. *Eur J Pediatr* 2005; 164: 648-9.
8. Renier WO. Compulsive spitting as manifestation of temporal lobe epilepsy. *Eur J Paediatr Neurol* 2004; 8: 61-2.
9. Fogarasi A, Janszky J, Siegler Z, Tuxhorn I. Ictal smile lateralizes to the right hemisphere in childhood epilepsy. *Epilepsia* 2005; 46: 449-51.
10. Fogarasi A, Janszky J, Tuxhorn I. Ictal pallor is associated with left temporal seizure onset zone in children. *Epilepsy Res* 2005; 67: 117-21.
11. Clarke DF, Otsubo H, Weiss SK, *et al*. The significance of ear plugging in localization-related epilepsy. *Epilepsia* 2003; 44: 1562-67.
12. Satow T, Ikeda A, Yamamoto J, *et al*. Partial epilepsy manifesting atonic seizure: report of two cases. *Epilepsia* 2002; 43: 1425-31.
13. Guzzetta F, Frisone MF, Ricci D, *et al*. Development of visual attention in West syndrome. *Epilepsia* 2002; 43: 757-3.
14. Eisermann M, Ville D, Soufflet C, *et al*. Cryptogenic Late Onset Epileptic Spasms: An Overlooked Syndrome of Early Childhood? *Epilepsia* 2006; 47: 1035-42.
15. Capovilla G, Beccaria F, Montagnini A. "Benign focal epilepsy in infancy with vertex spikes and waves during sleep". Delineation of the syndrome and recalling as "benign infantile focal epilepsy with midline spikes and waves during sleep" (BIMSE). *Brain Dev* 2006; 28: 85-91.
16. Zerr DM, Blume HK, Berg AT, *et al*. Nonfebrile illness seizures: a unique seizure category? *Epilepsia* 2005; 46: 952-5.
17. Sakai Y, Kira R, Torisu H *et al*. Benign convulsion with mild gastroenteritis and benign familial infantile seizure. *Epilepsy Res* 2006; 68: 269-71.
18. Heron SE, Crossland KM, Andermann E *et al*. Sodium-channel defects in benign familial neonatal-infantile seizures. *Lancet* 2002; 360: 851-2.
19. Striano P, Bordo L, Lispi ML, *et al*. A novel SCN2A mutation in family with benign familial infantile seizures. *Epilepsia* 2006; 47: 218-20.

20. Vanmolkot KR, Kors EE, Hottenga JJ, et al. Novel mutations in the Na+, K+-ATPase pump gene ATP1A2 associated with familial hemiplegic migraine and benign familial infantile convulsions. *Ann Neurol* 2003; 54: 360-6.
21. Teng D, Dayan P, Tyler S, et al. Risk of intracranial pathologic conditions requiring emergency intervention after a first complex febrile seizure episode among children. *Pediatrics* 2006; 117: 304-8.
22. Nabbout R, Prud'homme JF, Herman A, et al. A locus for simple pure febrile seizures maps to chromosome 6q22-q24. *Brain* 2002; 125: 2668-80.
23. Auvin S, Pandit F, De BJ, et al. Benign myoclonic epilepsy in infants: electroclinical features and long-term follow-up of 34 patients. *Epilepsia* 2006; 47: 387-93.
24. Mangano S, Fontana A, Cusumano L. Benign myoclonic epilepsy in infancy: neuropsychological and behavioural outcome. *Brain Dev* 2005; 27: 218-23.
25. Siegler Z, Barsi P, Neuwirth M, et al. Hippocampal sclerosis in severe myoclonic epilepsy in infancy: a retrospective MRI study. *Epilepsia* 2005; 46: 704-8.
26. Claes L, Del Favero J, Ceulemans B, et al. De novo mutations in the sodium-channel gene SCN1A cause severe myoclonic epilepsy of infancy. *Am J Hum Genet* 2001; 68: 1327-32.
27. Nabbout R, Gennaro E, Dalla BB, et al. Spectrum of SCN1A mutations in severe myoclonic epilepsy of infancy. *Neurology* 2003; 60: 1961-7.
28. Wallace RH, Hodgson BL, Grinton BE, et al. Sodium channel alpha1-subunit mutations in severe myoclonic epilepsy of infancy and infantile spasms. *Neurology* 2003; 61: 765-9.
29. Berkovic SF, Harkin LA, McMahon J, et al. De-novo mutations of the sodium channel gene SCN1A in alleged vaccine encephalopathy: a retrospective study. *Lancet Neurology* 2006.
30. Kimura K, Sugawara T, Mazaki-Miyazaki E, et al. A missense mutation in SCN1A in brothers with severe myoclonic epilepsy in infancy (SMEI) inherited from a father with febrile seizures. *Brain Dev* 2005; 27: 424-30.
31. Depienne C, Arzimanoglou A, Trouillard O, et al. Parental mosaicism can cause recurrent transmission of SCN1A mutations associated with severe myoclonic epilepsy of infancy. *Hum Mutat* 2006; 27.
32. Ceulemans BP, Claes LR, Lagae LG. Clinical correlations of mutations in the SCN1A gene: from febrile seizures to severe myoclonic epilepsy in infancy. *Pediatr Neurol* 2004; 30: 236-43.
33. Fujiwara T, Sugawara T, Mazaki-Miyazaki E, et al. Mutations of sodium channel alpha subunit type 1 (SCN1A) in intractable childhood epilepsies with frequent generalized tonic-clonic seizures. *Brain* 2003; 126: 531-46.
34. Nabbout R, Kozlovski A, Gennaro E, et al. Absence of mutations in major GEFS+ genes in myoclonic astatic epilepsy. *Epilepsy Res* 2003; 56: 127-33.
35. Monjauze C, Tuller L, Hommet C, et al. Language in benign childhood epilepsy with centrotemporal spikes abbreviated form: rolandic epilepsy and language. *Brain Lang* 2005; 92: 300-8.
36. Lindgren S, Kihlgren M, Melin L, et al. Development of cognitive functions in children with rolandic epilepsy. *Epilepsy Behav* 2004; 5: 903-10.
37. Vadlamudi L, Harvey AS, Connellan MM, et al. Is benign rolandic epilepsy genetically determined? *Ann Neurol* 2004; 56: 129-32.
38. Bast T, Volp A, Wolf C, Rating D. The influence of sulthiame on EEG in children with benign childhood epilepsy with centrotemporal spikes (BECTS). *Epilepsia* 2003; 44: 215-20.
39. Dubois CM, Zesiger P, Perez ER, et al. Acquired epileptic dysgraphia: a longitudinal study. *Dev Med Child Neurol* 2003; 45: 807-12.
40. Guerrini R, Sanchez-Carpintero R, Deonna T, et al. Early-onset absence epilepsy and paroxysmal dyskinesia. *Epilepsia* 2002; 43: 1224-9.
41. Auclair L, Jambaque I, Dulac O, et al. Deficit of preparatory attention in children with frontal lobe epilepsy. *Neuropsychologia* 2005; 43: 1701-12.
42. Lendt M, Gleissner U, Helmstaedter C, et al. Neuropsychological outcome in children after frontal lobe epilepsy surgery. *Epilepsy Behav* 2002; 3: 51-9.
43. Granata T, Gobbi G, Spreafico R, et al. Rasmussen's encephalitis: early characteristics allow diagnosis. *Neurology* 2003; 60: 422-5.

44. Chiapparini L, Granata T, Farina L, et al. Diagnostic imaging in 13 cases of Rasmussen's encephalitis: can early MRI suggest the diagnosis? *Neuroradiology* 2003; 45: 171-83.
45. Tobias SM, Robitaille Y, Hickey WF, et al. Bilateral Rasmussen encephalitis: postmortem documentation in a five-year-old. *Epilepsia* 2003; 44: 127-30.
46. Shah JR, Juhasz C, Kupsky WJ, et al. Rasmussen encephalitis associated with Parry-Romberg syndrome. *Neurology* 2003; 61: 395-7.
47. Watson R, Jiang Y, Bermudez I, et al. Absence of antibodies to glutamate receptor type 3 (GluR3) in Rasmussen encephalitis. *Neurology* 2004; 63: 43-50.
48. Bernasconi P, Cipelletti B, Passerini L, et al. Similar binding to glutamate receptors by Rasmussen and partial epilepsy patients' sera. *Neurology* 2002; 59: 1998-2001.
49. Bien, CG, Granata, T, Antozzi C, et al. Pathogenesis, diagnosis and treatment of Rasmussen encephalitis. A European consensus statement. *Brain* 2005; 128: 454-71.
50. Granata T, Fusco L, Gobbi G, et al. Experience with immunomodulatory treatments in Rasmussen's encephalitis. *Neurology* 2003; 61: 1807-10.
51. Lerman-Sagie T, Watemberg N, Vinkler C, et al. Familial hyperekplexia and refractory status epilepticus: a new autosomal recessive syndrome. *J Child Neurol* 2004; 19: 522-5.
52. Striano P, Boccella P, Sarappa C, Striano S. Spinal muscular atrophy and progressive myoclonic epilepsy: one case report and characteristics of the epileptic syndrome. *Seizure* 2004; 13: 582-6.
53. Haliloglu G, Chattopadhyay A, Skorodis L, et al. Spinal muscular atrophy with progressive myoclonic epilepsy: report of new cases and review of the literature. *Neuropediatrics* 2002; 33: 314-9.
54. Berg AT, Shinnar S, Testa FM, et al. Status epilepticus after the initial diagnosis of epilepsy in children. *Neurology* 2004; 63: 1027-34.
55. Chin RF, Verhulst L, Neville BG, et al. Inappropriate emergency management of status epilepticus in children contributes to need for intensive care. *J Neurol Neurosurg Psychiatry* 2004; 75: 1584-8.
56. Sillanpaa M, Shinnar S. Status epilepticus in a population-based cohort with childhood-onset epilepsy in Finland. *Ann Neurol* 2002; 52: 303-10.
57. Baxter P, Cross H, Livingstone J, et al. Idiopathic catastrophic childhood epileptic encephalopathy presenting with acute onset of intractable status. *Seizure* 2003.
58. Mikaeloff Y, Jambaque I, Hertz-Pannier L, et al. Devastating epileptic encephalopathy in school-age children (DESC): a pseudo-encephalitis. *Epilepsy Res* 2006; 69: 67-79.
59. Jambaque I, Hertz-Pannier L, Mikaeloff Y et al. Severe memory impairment in a child with bihippocampal injury after status epilepticus. *Dev Med Child Neurol* 2006; 48: 223-6.
60. Martins S, Guillery-Girard B, Jambaque I, et al. How children suffering severe amnesic syndrome acquire new concepts? *Neuropsychologia* 2006; 44: 2792-805.
61. Michelson-Kerman M, Watemberg N, Nissenkorn A, et al. Muscle glycogen depletion and increased oxidative phosphorylation following status epilepticus. *J Child Neurol* 2003; 18: 876-8.
62. Christiaens FJ, Mewasingh LD, Christophe C, et al. Unilateral cortical necrosis following status epilepticus with hypoglycemia. *Brain Dev* 2003; 25: 107-12.
63. Shah NS, Mitchell WG, Boles RG. Mitochondrial disorders: a potentially under-recognized etiology of infantile spasms. *J Child Neurol* 2002; 17: 369-72.
64. Desguerre I, Pinton F, Nabbout R, et al. Infantile spasms with basal ganglia MRI hypersignal may reveal mitochondrial disorder due to T8993G MT DNA mutation. *Neuropediatrics* 2003; 34: 265-9.
65. Sadleir LG, Connolly MB, Applegarth D, et al. Spasms in children with definite and probable mitochondrial disease. *Eur J Neurol* 2004; 11: 103-10.
66. Nguyen KV, Ostergaard E, Ravn SH, et al. POLG mutations in Alpers syndrome. *Neurology* 2005; 65: 1493-5.
67. Bahi-Buisson N, Kaminska A, Nabbout R., et al. Epilepsy in Menkes Disease: an original three step course. *Epilepsia* 2005; 47: 380-6.
68. Leary LD, Wang D, Nordli DR, Jr., et al. Seizure characterization and electroencephalographic features in Glut-1 deficiency syndrome. *Epilepsia* 2003; 44: 701-7.

69. Klepper J, Scheffer H, Leiendecker B, et al. Seizure control and acceptance of the ketogenic diet in GLUT1 deficiency syndrome: a 2- to 5-year follow-up of 15 children enrolled prospectively. *Neuropediatrics* 2005; 36: 302-8.
70. Mills PB, Struys E, Jakobs C, et al. Mutations in antiquitin in individuals with pyridoxine-dependent seizures. *Nat Med* 2006; 12: 307-9.
71. Mills PB, Surtees RA, Champion MP, et al. Neonatal epileptic encephalopathy caused by mutations in the PNPO gene encoding pyridox(am)ine 5'-phosphate oxidase. *Hum Mol Genet* 2005; 14: 1077-86.
72. Molinari F, Raas-Rothschild A, Rio M, et al. Impaired mitochondrial glutamate transport in autosomal recessive neonatal myoclonic epilepsy. *Am J Hum Genet* 2005; 76: 334-9.
73. Milh M, Becq H, Villeneuve N, Ben-Ari Y, Aniksztejn L. Inhibition of glutamate transporters results in a "suppression burst" pattern and partial seizure in the newborn rat. *Epilepsia* 2007; 48: 169-74.
74. Moretti P, Sahoo T, Hyland K, et al. Cerebral folate deficiency with developmental delay, autism, and response to folinic acid. *Neurology* 2005; 64: 1088-90.
75. Battaglia D, Zampino G, Zollino M, et al. Electroclinical patterns and evolution of epilepsy in the 4p- syndrome. *Epilepsia* 2003; 44: 1183-90.
76. Kagitani-Shimono K, Imai K, Otani K, et al. Epilepsy in Wolf-Hirschhorn syndrome (4p-). *Epilepsia* 2005; 46: 150-5.
77. Ville D, Kaminska A, Bahi-Buisson N, et al. Early pattern of epilepsy in the ring chromosome 20 syndrome. *Epilepsia* 2006; 47: 543-9.
78. Buoni S, Zannolli R, Colamaria V, et al. Myoclonic encephalopathy in the CDKL5 gene mutation. *Clin Neurophysiol* 2006; 117: 223-7.
79. Scala E, Ariani F, Mari F, et al. CDKL5/STK9 is mutated in Rett syndrome variant with infantile spasms. *J Med Genet* 2005; 42: 103-7.
80. Evans JC, Archer HL, Colley JP, et al. Early onset seizures and Rett-like features associated with mutations in CDKL5. *Eur J Hum Genet* 2005; 13: 1113-20.
81. Scheffer IE, Wallace RH, Phillips FL, et al. X-linked myoclonic epilepsy with spasticity and intellectual disability: mutation in the homeobox gene ARX. *Neurology* 2002; 59: 348-56.
82. Montenegro MA, Kinay D, Cendes F, et al. Patterns of hippocampal abnormalities in malformations of cortical development. *J Neurol Neurosurg Psychiatry* 2006; 77: 367-71.
83. Lortie A, Plouin P, Chiron C, et al. Characteristics of epilepsy in focal cortical dysplasia in infancy. *Epilepsy Res* 2002; 51: 133-45.
84. Fauser S, Schulze-Bonhage A. Epileptogenicity of cortical dysplasia in temporal lobe dual pathology: an electrophysiological study with invasive recordings. *Brain* 2006; 129: 82-95.
85. Sasaki M, Hashimoto T, Furushima W, et al. Clinical aspects of hemimegalencephaly by means of a nationwide survey. *J Child Neurol* 2005; 20: 337-41.
86. Salamon N, Andres M, Chute DJ, et al. Contralateral hemimicrencephaly and clinical-pathological correlations in children with hemimegalencephaly. *Brain* 2006; 129: 352-65.
87. Battaglia G, Chiapparini L, Franceschetti S, et al. Periventricular nodular heterotopia: classification, epileptic history, and genesis of epileptic discharges. *Epilepsia* 2006; 47: 86-97.
88. Wieck G, Leventer RJ, Squier WM, et al. Periventricular nodular heterotopia with overlying polymicrogyria. *Brain* 2005; 128: 2811-21.
89. Boudreau EA, Liow K, Frattali CM, et al. Hypothalamic hamartomas and seizures: distinct natural history of isolated and Pallister-Hall syndrome cases. *Epilepsia* 2005; 46: 42-7.
90. Harvey AS, Freeman JL, Berkovic SF, Rosenfeld JV. Transcallosal resection of hypothalamic hamartomas in patients with intractable epilepsy. *Epileptic Disord* 2003; 5: 257-65.
91. Delalande O, Fohlen M. Disconnecting surgical treatment of hypothalamic hamartoma in children and adults with refractory epilepsy and proposal of a new classification. *Neurol Med Chir (Tokyo)* 2003; 43: 61-8.
92. Kammoun F, Tanguy A, Boesplug-Tanguy O, et al. Club feet with congenital perisylvian polymicrogyria possibly due to bifocal ischemic damage of the neuraxis in utero. *Am J Med Genet A* 2004; 126: 191-6.
93. Chang BS, Piao X, Giannini C, et al. Bilateral generalized polymicrogyria (BGP): a distinct syndrome of cortical malformation. *Neurology* 2004; 62: 1722-8.

94. Chang BS, Piao X, Bodell A, et al. Bilateral frontoparietal polymicrogyria: clinical and radiological features in 10 families with linkage to chromosome 16. *Ann Neurol* 2003; 53: 596-606.
95. Lellouch-Tubiana A, Boddaert N, Bourgeois M, et al. Angiocentric neuroepithelial tumor (ANET): a new epilepsy-related clinicopathological entity with distinctive MRI. *Brain Pathol* 2005; 15: 281-6.
96. Trinka E, Unterrainer J, Haberlandt E, et al. Childhood febrile convulsions—which factors determine the subsequent epilepsy syndrome? A retrospective study. *Epilepsy Res* 2002; 50: 283-92.
97. Scott RC, King MD, Gadian DG, et al. Hippocampal abnormalities after prolonged febrile convulsion: a longitudinal MRI study. *Brain* 2003; 126: 2551-7.
98. Janszky J, Janszky I, Ebner A. Age at onset in mesial temporal lobe epilepsy with a history of febrile seizures. *Neurology* 2004; 63: 1296-8.
99. Terra-Bustamante VC, Inuzuca LM, Fernandes RM, et al. Temporal lobe epilepsy surgery in children and adolescents: clinical characteristics and post-surgical outcome. *Seizure* 2005; 14: 274-81.
100. Porter BE, Judkins AR, Clancy RR, et al. Dysplasia: a common finding in intractable pediatric temporal lobe epilepsy. *Neurology* 2003; 61: 365-8.
101. Clusmann H, Kral T, Gleissner U, et al. Analysis of different types of resection for pediatric patients with temporal lobe epilepsy. *Neurosurgery* 2004; 54: 847-59.
102. Goyal M, Bangert BA, Wiznitzer M. Mesial temporal sclerosis in acute childhood leukemias. *Epilepsia* 2003; 44: 131-4.
103. Madhyastha S, Somayaji SN, Rao MS, et al. Hippocampal brain amines in methotrexate-induced learning and memory deficit. *Can J Physiol Pharmacol* 2002; 80: 1076-84.
104. Major P, Decarie JC, Nadeau A, et al. Clinical significance of isolated hippocampal volume asymmetry in childhood epilepsy. *Neurology* 2004; 63: 1503-6.
105. Kobayashi E, Li LM, Lopes-Cendes I, Cendes F. Magnetic resonance imaging evidence of hippocampal sclerosis in asymptomatic, first-degree relatives of patients with familial mesial temporal lobe epilepsy. *Arch Neurol* 2002; 59: 1891-4.
106. Ng YT, McGregor AL, Wheless JW. Magnetic resonance imaging detection of mesial temporal sclerosis in children. *Pediatr Neurol* 2004; 30: 81-5.
107. Doherty MJ, Simon E, De Menezes MS, et al. When might hemispheric favouring of epileptiform discharges begin? *Seizure* 2003; 12: 595-8.
108. Chiron C, Jambaque I, Nabbout R, et al. The right brain hemisphere is dominant in human infants. *Brain* 1997; 120 (Pt 6): 1057-65.
109. Bahi-Buisson N, Kossorotoff M, Barnerias C, et al. Atypical case of hemiconvulsions-hemiplegia-epilepsy syndrome revealing contralateral focal cortical dysplasia. *Dev Med Child Neurol* 2005; 47: 830-4.
110. Mikaeloff Y, Jambaque I, Hertz-Pannier L, et al. Devastating epileptic encephalopathy in school-aged children (DESC): A pseudo encephalitis. *Epilepsy Res* 2006; 69: 67-79.
111. Camfield P, Camfield C, Lortie A, Darwish H. Infantile spasms in remission may reemerge as intractable epileptic spasms. *Epilepsia* 2003; 44: 1592-5.
112. Mitchell LA, Harvey AS, Coleman LT, et al. Anterior temporal changes on MR images of children with hippocampal sclerosis: an effect of seizures on the immature brain? *AJNR Am J Neuroradiol* 2003; 24: 1670-7.
113. Cohen I, Navarro V, Le DC, Miles R. Mesial temporal lobe epilepsy: a pathological replay of developmental mechanisms? *Biol Cell* 2003; 95: 329-33.
114. Cerminara C, Montanaro ML, Curatolo P, Seri S. Lamotrigine-induced seizure aggravation and negative myoclonus in idiopathic rolandic epilepsy. *Neurology* 2004; 63: 373-5.
115. McIntyre J, Robertson S, Norris E, et al. Safety and efficacy of buccal midazolam versus rectal diazepam for emergency treatment of seizures in children: a randomised controlled trial. *Lancet* 2005; 366: 205-10.
116. Baysun S, Aydin OF, Atmaca E, Gurer YK. A comparison of buccal midazolam and rectal diazepam for the acute treatment of seizures. *Clin Pediatr (Phila)* 2005; 44: 771-6.
117. Rainbow J, Browne GJ, Lam LT. Controlling seizures in the prehospital setting: diazepam or midazolam? *J Paediatr Child Health* 2002; 38: 582-6.

118. Bahi-Buisson N, Savini R, Eisermann M, *et al.* Misleading effects of clonazepam in symptomatic electrical status epilepticus during sleep syndrome. *Pediatr Neurol* 2006; 34: 146-50.
119. Elterman RD, Shields WD, Mansfield KA, Nakagawa J. Randomized trial of vigabatrin in patients with infantile spasms. *Neurology* 2001; 57: 1416-21.
120. Lux AL, Edwards SW, Hancock E, *et al.* The United Kingdom Infantile Spasms Study (UKISS) comparing hormone treatment with vigabatrin on developmental and epilepsy outcomes to age 14 months: a multicentre randomised trial. *Lancet Neurol* 2005; 4: 712-7.
121. Vanhatalo S, Nousiainen I, Eriksson K, *et al.* Visual field constriction in 91 Finnish children treated with vigabatrin. *Epilepsia* 2002; 43: 748-56.
122. Eisermann MM, de la Raillere A, Dellatolas G, *et al.* Infantile spasms in Down syndrome—effects of delayed anticonvulsive treatment. *Epilepsy Res* 2003; 55: 21-27.
123. Bergqvist AG, Schall JI, Gallagher PR, *et al.* Fasting versus gradual initiation of the ketogenic diet: a prospective, randomized clinical trial of efficacy. *Epilepsia* 2005; 46: 1810-9.
124. Feiz-Erfan I, Horn EM, Rekate HL, *et al.* Surgical strategies for approaching hypothalamic hamartomas causing gelastic seizures in the pediatric population: transventricular compared with skull base approaches. *J Neurosurg* 2005; 103: 325-32.
125. Delalande O, Fohlen M. Disconnecting surgical treatment of hypothalamic hamartoma in children and adults with refractory epilepsy and proposal of a new classification. *Neurol Med Chir (Tokyo)* 2003; 43: 61-8.
126. Cook SW, Nguyen ST, Hu B, *et al.* Cerebral hemispherectomy in pediatric patients with epilepsy: comparison of three techniques by pathological substrate in 115 patients. *J Neurosurg* 2004; 100: 125-41.
127. Bulteau C, Delalande O, Buret V, *et al.* Clinical results and long-term neuropsychological status after hemispherectomy. *Arch Pediatr* 2002; 9 Suppl 2: S90-91.
128. Yamamoto H, Yamano T, Niijima S, *et al.* Spontaneous improvement of intractable epileptic seizures following acute viral infections. *Brain Dev* 2004; 26: 377-9.
129. Bouma PA, Peters AC, Brouwer OF. Long term course of childhood epilepsy following relapse after antiepileptic drug withdrawal. *J Neurol Neurosurg Psychiatry* 2002; 72: 507-10.
130. Camfield P, Camfield C. The frequency of intractable seizures after stopping AEDs in seizure-free children with epilepsy. *Neurology* 2005; 64: 973-5.

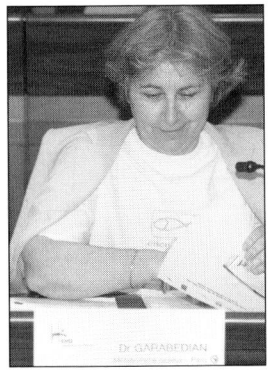

Calcium, Phosphorus, and Metabolic Bone Diseases in Children: What has Changed over the Past Five Years

Michèle GARABÉDIAN

INSERM U561, Saint Vincent de Paul Hospital, Paris, France

Although no decisive changes have recently emerged for the management of children with bone diseases, the last five years have seen several major breakthroughs in the understanding of bone and phosphate metabolism that open new perspectives for the diagnosis and treatment of these diseases. Key genes have been identified as the causes of classical bone diseases, especially hypophosphatemia rickets and osteomalacia. Other genes have enriched the list of the genetic defects responsible for osteoporosis or, inversely, for high bone density and osteopetrosis. Several of these identifications, in association with animal studies and the development of new biological tools, have drastically modified and enriched our operating models for phosphate homeostasis and for the coupling of bone formation/resorption. Moreover, they open the way to new therapeutic strategies. Progress concerning calcium metabolism have not been so crucial. However, despite recent controversies, most epidemiological and interventional studies confirm the importance of dietary calcium for bone growth during childhood, and new genes have been identified that control parathyroid glands and target cell responses to parathyroid hormone. Details of these advances are presented below, with special emphasis on studies related to children and adolescents.

What has recently changed in our knowledge of metabolic bone diseases

At the turn of this century, numerous gene defects had been identified as responsible for major hereditary bone diseases, like osteogenesis imperfecta (type I collagens), achondroplasia and hypochondroplasia (*FGFR3*), dominant craniosynostosis (*FGFR2*), the Leri-Weill syndrome (*SHOX*), pycnodysostosis (cathepsin K), Marfan syndrome (fibrillin-1), the congenital contractural arachnodactyly (fibrillin-2), and the multiple exostoses syndrome (*EXT1* and *EXT2*). Further works during the past five years have led to the discovery of other genetic defects that not only enable the genetic diagnosis of additional bone diseases, but also improve our understanding of bone metabolism.

In parallel, new tools have been added to the cluster of biological markers of bone metabolism, aside from the usual serum and/or urinary assays of bone formation (osteocalcin, alkaline phosphatase activity) and bone resorption (tartrate resistant acid phosphatase activity and degradation products of type I collagen). The serum assay of these new markers, RANK-L and osteoprotegerin, theoretically explores the coupling between bone formation and resorption (see below). But their interest in general practice remains to be evaluated, as measured levels in children appear to reflect compensatory responses to bone loss rather than its causal mechanism [1].

As for the therapeutic approaches, the development of new classes of bisphosphonates with considerably higher activity on bone resorption have brought definite improvement in the management of hyperresorptive osteoporosis in children [2]. Patients with severe hypercalcemia, caused by malignancy or hyperparathyroidism, and patients with osteogenesis imperfecta have been the first to benefit from these treatments. However, other patients with bone diseases secondary to, or aggravated by, excessive bone resorption, experience a decreased rate of fractures, diminished bone pain, and increased bone mass, under treatment. These are patients with long term immobilization, Paget's disease or idiopathic hyperphosphatasia, steroid-induced osteoporosis, or localized bone defects like in the McCune-Albright syndrome. At the same time, bone anabolic drugs are currently being tested for the treatment of osteoporosis, mainly teriparatide, the human 1-34 parathyroid hormone, while other ways of stimulating the osteoblast lineage are being explored, via activation of the Wnt/*LRP5* pathway for example (see below).

Newly identified genes involved in diseases of bone formation

The recent multiplication of putative causal gene defects obfuscate the cause of some bone diseases. For example, dominant types of multiple epiphyseal dysplasia which were thought to result from defects in type IX collagen genes (*COL9A1, COL9A2, COL9A3*), have now been associated with defects in three additional genes coding for extracellular matrix proteins of the cartilage, namely the oligomeric matrix protein (COMP), DTDST, and matrilin-3 (MATN3). Moreover, a recent screening failed to detect a genetic cause in about half of the patients, suggesting that several other protein defects in the growth plate cartilage matrix may cause the disease [3].

In contrast, discoveries of mutations in genes coding for major regulatory factors of the osteoblast lineage have confirmed the key role played by these factors in bone formation, unveiled the cause of several hereditary bone diseases, and added new causal or aggravating factors of osteoporosis (*table I*).

The first of these factors, *TGF-beta1*, controls osteoblast proliferation and differentiation. Gene mutations in the signal peptide and in the latency-associated peptide (beta1-LAP) of *TGF-beta1*, that activate this transforming growth factor, are responsible for the progressive hyperosteosis and diaphyseal dysplasia of Camurati-Engelman [4].

The second factor, the core binding factor A1 (*CBF A1/RUNX2*), plays a key role in early osteoblast differentiation and chondrocyte maturation. Mutations in this gene have not only been identified in patients with the dominantly inherited cleidocranial dysplasia associating open skull sutures and clavicular hypoplasia, but also in patients with supernumerary teeth, and/or in patients with osteoporosis and fractures [5]. Moreover, polymorphic variants of this gene have been associated with bone mineral density in women and with the risk for Colle's fracture in the elderly [6]. Finally, studies in transgenic null-mice suggest that another factor of the runt-family (*CBF beta*) may also be involved in bone development and occurrence of cleido-cranial dysplasia [7].

The third factor is the low-density lipoprotein receptor related protein 5 (LRP5) expressed in osteoblasts and regions of bone remodeling. In association with other

Table I. Recently identified causal genes related to bone or phospho-calcic metabolic diseases in children.

Gene	Disease	Authors
Related to bone diseases		
CBF A1 (and CBFbeta)	Cleidocranial dysplasia, teeth anomalies, osteoporosis	Qack 1999 [5], Kundu 2002 [7]
TGF beta 1	Camurati-Engelman syndrome	Janssens 2006 [4]
LRP5 (loss-of-function)	Osteoporosis/pseudoglioma Juvenile osteoporosis	Gong 2001 [8] Hartikka 2005 [9]
LRP5 (gain-of-function)	Autosomal dominant high bone density	Boyden 2002 [10]
TCIRG1	Infantile malignant osteopetrosis	Frattini 2000 [31]
C1CN7 (chloride channel)	Dominant and recessive osteopetrosis	Cleiren 2001 [32]
TNFRSF11B (osteoprotegerin)	Idiopathic hyperphosphatasia	Cundy 2002 [13]
TNFRSF11A (RANK)	Idiopathic hyperphosphatasia	Daroszewska 2005 [15]
MATN3 (matrilin-3)	Multiple epiphyseal dysplasia	Chapman 2001 [33]
SH3BP2	Cherubism	Ueki 2001 [34]
Related to calcium metabolism		
HRPT2 (parafibromin)	Hyperparathyroidism-jaw tumour syndrome	Carpten 2002 [35]
TBCE	Kenny Caffey/HRD	Parvari 2002 [22]
TBX1	Del22q11 syndrome	Yagi 2003 [23]
GCMB	Hypoparathyroidism	Ding 2001 [36]
STX16	PHP1b	Bastepe 2003 [25]
Related to Phosphate metabolism		
PHEX	Hypophosphatemic rickets	Rowe 2004 (review) [26]
FGF23 (stabilization)	Hypophosphatemic rickets	White 2005 (review) [27]
FGF23 (destabilization)	Familial tumoural calcinosis	White 2005 (review) [27]
Na-Pi 2a	Hypophosphatemia, hypercalciuria, and osteoporosis	Prie 2002 [30]
SLC34A3 (Na-Pi 2c)	Hypophosphatemic rickets with hypercalciuria	Lorenz-Depiereux 2006 [29] Bergwitz 2006 [28]

proteins, it forms receptor complexes that bind Wnt glycoproteins, thus initiating a cascade of events leading to the translocation of beta-catenin into the nucleus and to its effects on gene expression. The regulatory role of the LRP5/Wnt pathway on bone accrual during growth has been clearly unveiled by findings of loss-of-function LRP5 mutations in the rare patients presenting with the osteoporosis-pseudoglioma syndrome [8] and in a few patients with juvenile and adult osteoporosis [9]. Inversely, patients with dominantly inherited high bone mass, associated or not with craniosynostosis or oropharyngeal exostoses, have been shown to present gain-of-function mutations in LRP5 that increase Wnt signaling by reducing the inhibitory activity of the DKK-1 protein on the Wnt pathway [10]. Association studies in healthy cohorts also suggest some contribution of the LRP5 genotype to variability in bone mineral density in the general population [11].

Newly identified genes controlling bone resorption

Similarly, the identification of new gene mutations in patients with osteopetrosis has confirmed the key role played by these genes in osteoclast functions and greatly facilitated the genetic diagnosis of the disease. Unlike in osteopetrotic mice, osteopetrosis in humans results from a defective function of the osteoclast rather than from a deficient production of these cells. Mutations in the Carbonic Anhydrase II gene (*CA2*) alter both the osteoclast and renal tubular functions and are classically observed in patients whose features associate autosomic recessive osteopetrosis, tubular acidosis and intracerebral calcifications. Two other genes account for the majority of the osteopetrotic cases in humans, *C1CN7* and *TCIRG1* (*Table I*). They encode the *C1CN7* chloride channel and the a3 subunit of the vacuolar proton pump respectively, and thus locally influence the osteoclast activity of bone resorption. Nearly 60% of the patients with a recessive infantile malignant osteopetrosis (ARO) bear *TCIRG1* mutations, while mutations in the *C1CN7* gene are found in all patients with the less severe dominant adult form (*ADO II*). Yet, *C1CN7* mutations on one or two alleles have also been reported in some infants with the severe form (13%), and large variations in the clinical manifestations linked to *C1CN7* mutations, even within the same family, complicate prenatal diagnosis [12].

Newly identified genes and new concepts to understand the coupling between bone formation and resorption

A major leap forward the understanding of the coupling between bone formation and resorption has been the recent description of the RANK/RANK-L/osteoprotegerin system (*figure 1*). RANK-L is produced by the osteoblasts and activates osteoclastogenesis by binding to the RANK protein (Receptor Activating the NF Kappa B system) expressed at the surface of pre-osteoclasts. Osteoprotegerin is also produced by osteoblasts but acts as a soluble decoy receptor for RANK-L, thus decreasing its availability to bind RANK and hence, its stimulatory effect on osteoclast functions. Findings of deactivating mutations in the osteoprotegerin gene (*TNFRSF11B*) offer a valuable explanation to the abnormally high bone turn-over found in patients with idiopathic juvenile hyperphosphatasia [13]. Further studies have confirmed the importance of this system by showing associations between osteoprotegerin gene variants and the risk of developing Paget's diseases of bone, although other causal genes, like Sequestosome 1, are known to be involved in the classical form of Paget's disease [14]. Moreover, activating mutations in the RANK gene (*TNFRSF11 A*) itself have been identified in patients with familial expansile osteolysis, and in some cases of infantile Paget's diseases and familial expansile skeletal hyperphosphatasia [15]. However, no human disease has been identified yet involving defects in the *TNFSF11* gene encoding RANK-L.

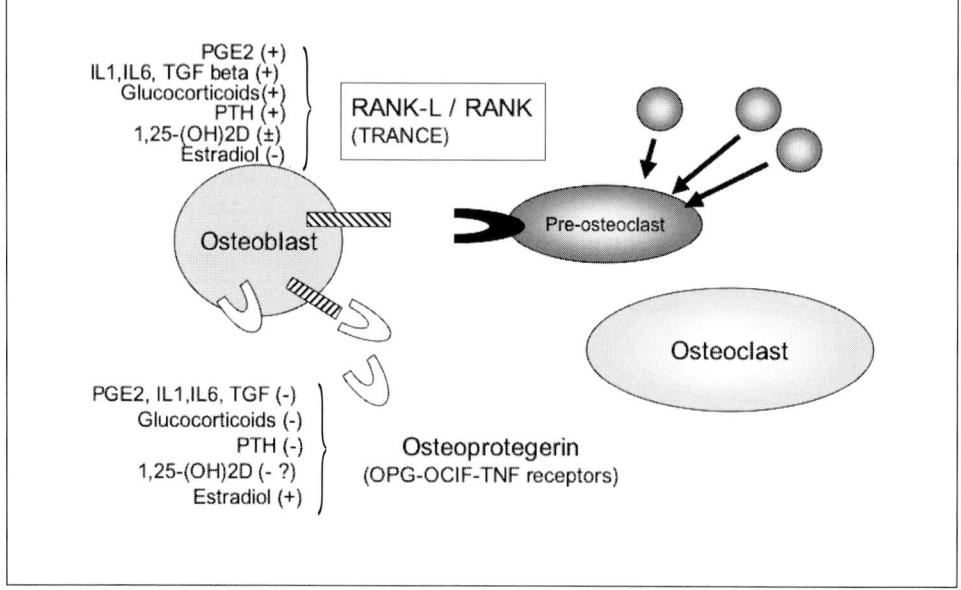

Figure 1. Bone formation-resorption coupling.

What has changed in diseases of calcium metabolism

Recent changes in this domain concern new therapeutic approaches of hyperparathyroidism and the unveiling of further genes at the origin of parathyroid dysfunctions. Also, and despite recent controversies related to the importance of dietary calcium for bone growth and mineralization [16-18], an extensive survey of healthy women bring forth strong evidence for a deleterious effect of deficient milk consumption during childhood on fracture risk in women before and after 50 year of age [19].

Several new analogs of vitamin D have been recently developed, some of them putatively more specifically active on bone or parathyroid over-activity than the widely used 1.25-dihydroxyvitamin D3, but with less hypercalcemic effect. But clinical trials are still in progress and their beneficial effects remain uncertain. In contrast, the identification of the Calcium sensing receptor (CasR) as a key step in the control of parahyroid secretion has initiated the development of "calcimimetic" drugs that up-regulates CasR and thus amplify the inhibitory effect of calcium on the production of parathyroid hormone [20]. These drugs are currently evaluated in adult patients with primary or secondary hyperparathyroidism and their use in paediatric nephrology is beginning.

Primary hyperparathyroidism is seldom observed in children, but the choice of its management, surgical or medical, must consider the cause of the disease. This may be easy when hyperparathyroidism is part of a known syndrome (familial hypocalciuric-hyercalcaemia, multiple endocrine neoplasia, hyperparathyroidism-jaw tumour syndrome). However, cases of isolated hyperparathyroidism, especially when multiglandular, may require genotyping of the patients (MEN 1, CaSR), although genetic testing have been negative in 60% of the patients with familial isolated hyperparathyroidism [21].

Hypoparathyroidism is more frequent in children. Progress in this domain has been limited to the identification of a few causal genes (*Table 1*). Particularly, it has been found that patients with Kenny-Caffey (MIM24460) and patients with Sanjad-Sakati or HRD (MIM24410) syndromes bear a genetic defect in the *TBCE* gene, encoding a chaperone protein involved in the tubulin assembly pathway. This suggests that a common pathophysiological mechanism is responsible for these two, and so far distinct, autosomal recessive syndromes associating congenital hypoparathyroidism, growth and mental retardation and a characteristic physiognomy [22]. In addition, the DiGeorge syndrome, conotruncal anomaly face syndrome and velocardiofacial syndrome are frequent microdeletion syndromes known since long to be associated with 22q11.2 deletions. But more than 30 genes have been mapped to the deleted region and the causal gene defect(s) remained unknown. Identification of mutations in the *TBX1* gene in patients with these syndromes but no 22q11.2 deletion, strongly suggests that *TBX1* is a major determinant of the 22q11.2 deletion syndrome and is a decisive step towards a better understanding of these syndromes and diagnosis accuracy [23].

Finally, important advances have been made in the comprehension of parathyroid resistances. The classical type of resistance to parathyroid hormone (PHP-1a), associated with features of Albright osteodystrophy including heterotopic ossifications (AHO), is since long known to result from defects in the *GNAS1* gene. Inactivating mutations in *GNAS1* lead to defective activity of the alpha subunit of the Gs protein and, hence, to decreased response to parathyroid hormone. The phenotypes associated with this gene defect have now been extended to cases of isolated extra-osseous calcifications, osteoma cutis and progressive osseous heteroplasia, suggesting the importance of the Gs/AMPc pathway for the control of osteoblast formation [24]. Moreover, there is now clear evidence for a maternal transmission of the parathyroid hormone resistance via imprinting of *GNAS1* in the proximal tubule, while such imprinting likely does not occur in the other target cells. The specific loss of *GNAS1* expression in the renal proximal tubule induces another maternally transmitted type of parathyroid hormone resistance (PHP-1b), not associated with AHO features. It has been associated with deletions within *STX16*, a closely linked gene centromeric of *GNAS1* which encodes syntaxin-16 and contains a cis-acting element that controls imprinting of the maternal GNAS allele [25].

What has changed in diseases of phosphate metabolism

Major advances in this field occured during the last five years. They have greatly changed our conception of phosphate homeostasis and initiated stimulating openings towards improved diagnosis and management of phosphate disorders. Ten years ago, defects in the PHEX gene have been identified as the cause of X-linked hypophosphatemic rickets, the most common form of hereditary of rickets. Shortly thereafter, tumour-induced hypophosphatemia was found to result from an abnormal local production of a growth factor, FGF 23, and mutations in the gene encoding this factor that increase the stability of the peptide, and its circulating concentration, were found in patients with ADHR, an autosomal dominant inherited hypophosphatemic bone disease [26, 27]. Inversely, FGF 23 mutations causing destabilization of the peptide have been identified in some patients with hyperphosphatemia and familial tumoral calcinosis. Moreover, gene defects in two genes encoding renal transporters of phosphate, the Na-Pi-2c and the Na-Pi-2a, have been found in patients with familial hypophosphatemia rickets and hypercalciuria [28, 29], and in adult hypophosphatemic patients with osteoporosis [30] respectively.

These findings and ensuing animal and *in vitro* studies, as well as the development of FGF23 and MEPE assays in serum, have considerably enlighten our view of the control of phosphate homeostasis (*figure 2*). Briefly, a new set of factors, named "phosphatonins", are now considered to be key regulatory factors of serum phosphate, aside from parathyroid hormone, which regulates serum phosphate via bone resorption and renal tubular reabsorption, and from calcitriol, which mainly acts at the intestinal level. These phosphatonins inhibit the sodium-phosphate transporters in the proximal convoluted tubules, thus decreasing serum phosphate, and decrease the production of 1.25-(OH) 2D3, thus decreasing the ability of the intestine to absorb phosphate. At least, three hypophosphatemic factors have been identified from tumours: the secreted frizzled protein 4, MEPE, a matrix extracellular phosphoglycoprotein expressed in odontoblasts and osteocytes embedded in mineralized matrix, and FGF 23, mainly expressed in regions of active bone formation and remodelling. High phosphate diet, elevated serum phosphate levels, as well as 1.25-(OH) 2D, increase FGF 23 secretion, which in turn decreases serum phosphate and vitamin D levels and thus protects the organism against the deleterious effects of excessive phosphate levels. This phosphate feed-back mechanism is less operative in conditions of low serum calcium, thus decreasing the risk of hypocalcemia. PHEX is also expressed in osteoblasts and odontoblasts and encodes a protease that probably interacts with circulating phosphatonins. But PHEX ligands remain unknown, although PHEX mutations have been associated with increased levels of FGF23 and of the MEPE/ASARM-peptide. In any case, FGF23 appears to be responsible for the low serum phosphate and 1.25-(OH) 2D levels observed in patients with either PHEX mutations, FGF23 mutations that stabilize the peptide, or phosphatonin producing tumours. These findings provide new possible strategies to treat hypophosphatemic diseases and to reduce hyperphosphatemia in renal insufficiency, using for instance FGF23 antibodies or antagonists, or FGF23 analogs.

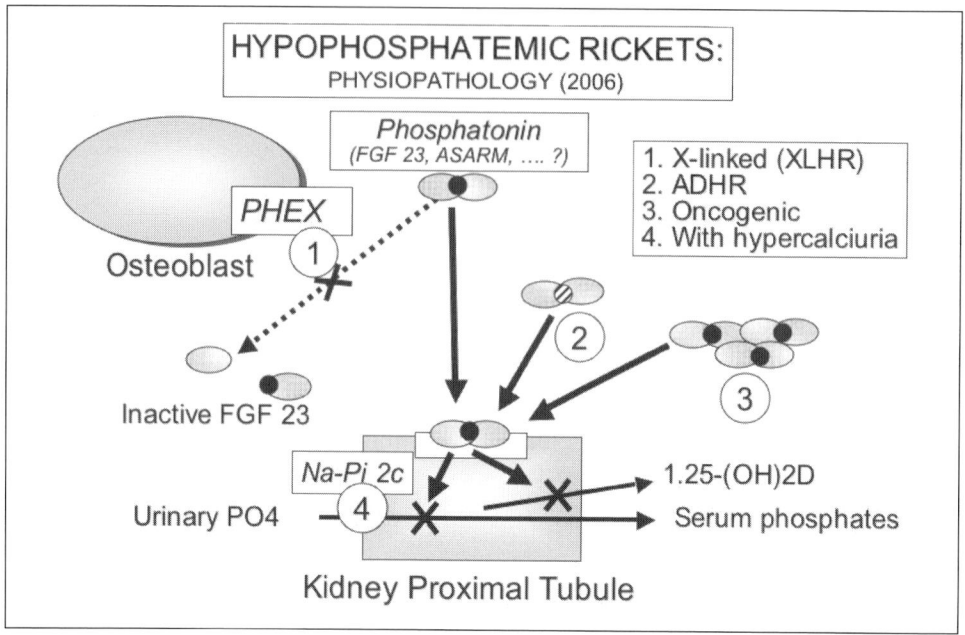

Figure 2. Control of phospate homeostasis.

References

1. Misra M, Soyka LA, Miller KK, et al. Serum osteoprotegerin in adolescent girls with anorexia nervosa. *J Clin Endocrinol Metab* 2003; 88: 3816-22.
2. Srivastava T, Alon US. The role of bisphosphonates in diseases of childhood. *Eur J Pediatr* 2003; 162: 735-51.
3. Itoh T, Shirahama S, Nakashima E, et al. Comprehensive screening of multiple epiphyseal dysplasia mutations in Japanese population. *Am J Med Genet* 2006; 15: 1280-4.
4. Janssens K, Vanhoenacker F, Bonduelle M, et al. Camurati-Engelmann disease: review of the clinical, radiological, and molecular data of 24 families and implications for diagnosis and treatment. *J Med Genet* 2006; 43: 1-11.
5. Quack I, Vonderstrass B, Stock M, et al. Mutation analysis of core binding factor A1 in patients with cleidocranial dysplasia. *Am J Hum Genet* 1999; 65: 1268-78.
6. Vaughan T, Pasco JA, Kotowicz MA, et al. Alleles of RUNX2/CBFA1 gene are associated with differences in bone mineral density and risk of fracture. *J Bone Miner Res* 2002; 17: 1527-34.
7. Kundu M, Javed A, Jeon JP, et al. CBFbeta interacts with Runx2 and has a critical role in bone development. *Nat Genet* 2002; 32: 639-44.
8. Gong Y, Slee RB, Fukai N, et al. for the Osteoporosis-Pseudoglioma Syndrome Collaborative Group. LDL-receptor-related protein 5 (LRP5) affects bone accrual and eye development. *Cell* 2001; 107: 513-23.
9. Hartikka H, Makitie O, Mannikko M, et al. Heterozygous mutations in the LDL receptor-related protein 5 (LRP5) gene are associated with primary osteoporosis in children. *J Bone Miner Res* 2005; 20: 783-9.

10. Boyden LM, Mao J, Belsky J, et al. High bone density due to mutation in LDL-receptor-related protein 5. *N Engl J Med* 2002; 16: 1513-21.
11. Koay MA, Woon PY, Zhang Y, et al. Influence of LRP5 polymorphisms on normal variation in BMD. *J Bone Miner Res* 2004; 19: 1619-27.
12. Frattini A, Pangrazio A, Susani L, et al. Chloride channel ClCN7 mutations are responsible for severe recessive, dominant, and intermediate osteopetrosis. *J Bone Miner Res* 2003; 18: 1740-7.
13. Cundy T, Hegde M, Naot D, et al. A mutation in the gene TNFRSF11B encoding osteoprotegerin causes an idiopathic hyperphosphatasia phenotype. *Hum Mol Genet* 2002; 11: 2119-27.
14. Daroszewska A, Hocking LJ, McGuigan FE, et al. Susceptibility to Paget's disease of bone is influenced by a common polymorphic variant of osteoprotegerin. *J Bone Miner Res* 2004; 19: 1506-11.
15. Daroszewska A, Ralston SH. Genetic of Paget's disease of bone. *Clin Sci* 2005; 109: 257-63.
16. Heaney RP. Calcium, dairy products and osteoporosis. *J Am Coll Nutr* 2000; 19: S83-S99.
17. Weinsier RL, Krumdieck CL. Dairy foods and bone health: examination of the evidence. *Am J Clin Nutr* 2000; 72: 681-9.
18. Lanou AJ, Berkow SE, Barnard ND. Calcium, dairy products, and bone health in children and young adults: a reevaluation of the evidence. *Pediatrics* 2005; 115: 736-43.
19. Kalkwarf HJ, Khoury JC, Lanphear BP. Milk intake during childhood and adolescence, adult bone density, and osteoporotic fractures in US women. *Am J Clin Nutr* 2003; 77: 257-65.
20. Quarles LD. Cinacalcet HCl: a novel treatment for secondary hyperparathyroidism in stage 5 chronic kidney disease. *Kidney* 2005; 96: S24-8.
21. Warner J, Epstein M, Sweet A, et al. Genetic testing in familial isolated hyperparathyroidism: unexpected results and their implications. *J Med Genet* 2004; 41: 155-60.
22. Parvari R, Hershkovitz E, Grossman N, et al. HRD/Autosomal Recessive Kenny-Caffey Syndrome Consortium. Mutation of TBCE causes hypoparathyroidism-retardation-dysmorphism and autosomal recessive Kenny-Caffey syndrome. *Nat Genet* 2002; 32: 448-52.
23. Yagi H, Furutani Y, Hamada H, et al. Role of TBX1 in human del22q11.2 syndrome. *Lancet* 2003; 362: 1366-73.
24. Yeh GL, Mathur S, Wivel A, et al. GNAS1 mutation and Cbfa1 misexpression in a child with severe congenital platelike osteoma cutis. *J Bone Miner Res* 2000; 15: 2063-73.
25. Bastepe M, Fröhlich LF, Hendry GN, et al. Autosomal dominant pseudohydroparathyroidism type Ib is associated with heterozygous microdeletion that likely disrupts a putative imprinting control element of GNAS. *J Clin Invest* 2003; 112: 1255-63.
26. Rowe PS. The wrickkened pathways of FGF23, MEPE and PHEX. *Crit Rev Oral Biol Med* 2004; 15: 264-81.
27. White KE, Larsson TM, Econs MJ. The roles of specific genes implicated as circulating factors involved in normal and disordered phosphate homeostasis: Frp-4, MEPE, and FGF 23. *Endocrine Reviews* 2006; 3: 221-41.
28. Bergwitz C, Roslin NM, Tieder M, et al. SLC34A3 Mutations in patients with hereditary hypophosphatemic rickets with hypercalciuria predict a key role for the sodium-phosphate cotransporter napi-iic in maintaining phosphate homeostasis. *Am J Hum Genet* 2006; 78: 179-92.
29. Lorenz-Depiereux B, Benet-Pages A, Eckstein G, et al. Hereditary hypophosphatemic rickets with hypercalciuria is caused by mutations in the sodium-phosphate cotransporter gene SLC34A3. *Am J Hum Genet* 2006; 78: 193-201.
30. Prie D, Huart V, Bakouh N, et al. Nephrolithiasis and osteoporosis associated with hypophosphatemia caused by mutations in the type 2a sodium-phosphate cotransporter. *N Engl J Med* 2002; 347: 983-91.
31. Frattini A, Orchard PJ, Sobacchi C, et al. Defects in TCIRG1 subunit of the vacuolar proton pump are responsible for a subset of human autosomal recessive osteopetrosis. *Nat Genet* 2000; 25: 343-6.
32. Cleiren E, Benichou O, Van Hul E, et al. Albers-Schonberg disease (autosomal dominant osteopetrosis, type II) results from mutations in the ClCN7 chloride channel gene. *Hum Mol Genet* 2001; 10: 2861-7.

Genetics

Congenital nephrotic syndrome

The term *congenital nephrotic syndrome* (CNS) applies to a nephrotic syndrome (NS) present at birth or developing during the first 3 months of life. Most of the CNSs have a genetic basis, and a poor outcome. Recent progress in molecular genetics and biology has given new insights into the molecular basis of the different forms of CNS [1]. The CNSs are usually classified as primary CNS or acquired CNS (syphilis, toxoplasmosis, rubella, CMV, hepatitis B, HIV).

The primary forms of CNS are most often genetically determined. The genes and their mutations responsible for CNS have been identified:
– CNS of Finnish type: the gene *NPHS1* has been localized on chromosome 19, and its product, nephrin, identified. The integrity of nephrin is crucial for the formation and maintenance of the slit diaphragms and podocytes in the glomerulus. *NPHS1* inactivation in mice leads to massive proteinuria, disappearance of the podocyte foot processes, absence of slit diaphragms and neonatal death [2].
– Mutations of the gene *NPHS2* have been observed in autosomal recessive steroid-resistant NS. Prenatal diagnosis is based on the analysis of *NPHS2* in placental or amniotic fluid cells of at risk fetuses. Rapid antenatal screening is possible because of the small size of the gene.
– Denys-Drash syndrome is a rare condition associating nephropathy, male pseudo-hermaphrodism and Wilms tumour. This syndrome is due to mutations of the gene *WT1*.
– The gene *LMX1B* encodes a transcription factor expressed in the podocytes from the early stages of differentiation. Mutation of this gene may be responsible for the congenital forms of NS sometimes associated with the nail-patella syndrome [3].

Nephronophthisis

Nephronophthisis (NPH) is an autosomal recessive kidney disease that leads to end-stage renal failure in the first two decades of life. Following the pioneering work of Antignac et al., [4] and that of Hildebrandt et al., [5] several genes and gene products have been identified in the various forms of nephronophthisis [6]: *NPHP1* and *nephrocystin*; *NPHP2* and *inversin*; *NPHP3* and *nephrocystin-3*; *NPHP4* and *nephroretinin*. Mutations in the gene *NPHP5*, encoding for *nephrocystin-5* are present in the renal-retinal Senior-Loken syndrome.

Primary hyperoxaluria type 1

It is due to the deficiency of the liver-specific enzyme alanine: glyoxylate aminotransferase (AGT). The AGT gene (*AGXT*) is a single gene copy which maps to chromosome 2q37.3. More than 65 mutations in the gene *AGXT* have been identified so far [7]. Prenatal diagnosis using a combination of linked polymorphism and detection of the two most common mutations has an accuracy of more than 99% and can be performed on chorionic villi or amniocytes [8]. Several missense, nonsense, and deletion mutations in the gene responsible for primary hyperoxaluria type 2 (*GRHPR*) encoding glyoxylate reductase (GR) and for hydroxyl-pyruvate-reductase (HPR) have also been recently identified [9].

Miscellaneous hereditary tubulopathies

Remarkable progress has been made in the understanding of the molecular pathogenesis of various congenital tubulopathies. Loss-of-function or gain-of-function mutations in genes encoding channel, cotransporter or exchanger proteins located in the luminal, basolateral, or endosomal cell membranes have been described. These mutations result in a variety of functional defects. A basic science review has summarized valuable information on this topic [10].

Assessment of glomerular filtration rate (GFR)

In children, GFR is commonly assessed by measuring the urinary clearance of endogenous creatinine. To avoid the need for urinary collection, formulae have been developed based on the ratio of the patient's height (as reflecting muscle mass and hence creatinine production) to the plasma creatinine. The so-called Schwartz and Counahan-Barratt formulae provide the paediatrician with reasonable estimates of GFR.

In the mid-eighties, cystatin C was proposed as a new endogenous marker of GFR. It was later claimed to be a better marker than creatinine, because its plasma concentration did not appear to be influenced by gender, lean tissue mass and inflammation [11, 12]. As it is filtered and completely reabsorbed by the renal tubules, cystatin C is not a standard marker of GFR, and its urinary clearance can obviously not be measured.

Most studies have tried to validate cystatin C using common markers of GFR such as creatinine clearance, or the plasma clearance of edetic acid or iohexol. Very few studies have used the gold standard, that is the urinary clearance of inulin, for the validation of cystatin C. A major clinical recent study in adults has clearly shown that male gender, older age, greater weight, higher serum C-reactive-protein-levels, and cigarette smoking, are all independently associated with higher serum concentrations of cystatin C after adjusting for creatinine clearance [13]. Cystatin C has also been shown to be a poor marker of GFR in renal transplant patients and/or in patients receiving steroids [14, 15]. In a recent study in children, using the urinary clearance of inulin as the gold standard, cystatin C has been shown to be less reliable than the Schwartz formula in distinguishing impaired from normal GFR [16]. The cost effectiveness of cystatin C is extremely low, its measurement being 12 times more expensive than that of creatinine [11]. Contrary to the claim, cystatin C does not appear to be a better marker of GFR than creatinine and its routine use cannot be recommended.

Management of renal diseases

Nephrotic syndrome

Most children presenting with minimal changes idiopathic NS respond to steroids. A third of them develop frequent relapses, requiring the use of large toxic doses of steroids. Alternative immunosuppressive regimens have been tried, including i.v. methylprednisolone, triamcinolone, oral and parenteral cyclophosphamide, cyclosporine, tacrolimus, and levamisole.

Cyclophosphamide is often used in frequent relapsers. It is efficient but may induce neutropenia, as well as bladder and gonadal damage. Cyclosporin is also effective but may have adverse nephrotoxic effects and cause hypertension. Cyclosporine is mostly used in steroid-dependent as well as in steroid-resistant forms of NS. Because of the side effects of steroids, calcineurin-inhibitors and cyclophosphamide, there is clearly often a need for alternative immunosuppressive drugs.

Mycophenolate mofetil (MMF) is a selective reversible inhibitor of inosine-monophosphate-dehydrogenase that inhibits the "*de novo*" synthesis of purines. It appears to represent an interesting adjunctive therapy for NS. In a few studies in children with steroid-dependent or steroid-resistant NS previously treated with prednisone, levamisole and/or cyclophosphamide, MMF resulted in a steroid-sparing effect, with consequent improvement in growth velocity, physical appearance and blood pressure [17, 18]. This allowed significant reductions in the dose of steroids required to control the disease. The beneficial effect of MMF has been confirmed in a recent prospective study in children with steroid-dependent NS [19]. The beneficial effects of MMF were obtained with a daily target dose of 600 mg/m^2. This regimen was associated with only mild side effects, gastrointestinal discomfort being usually self-limited.

The profile of MMF, its potential for a virtual cure in some children, and its therapeutic benefit in most children, argue in favour of using this product as the first line adjunctive therapy for steroid-dependent nephrotic syndromes. Randomized clinical trials are clearly needed to define clinical guidelines for an optimal use of MMF [20]. In children treated with the standard oral glucocorticoid protocol, relapses are frequently due to non-compliance. In these patients, the use of steroids with prolonged half-life such as triamcinolone-acetonide can be helpful [21].

Chronic renal failure

Anaemia

Recombinant human erythropoietin (rHuEPO) increases hemoglobin and reduces the need for blood transfusion in patients with chronic renal failure. While the intravenous administration of erythropoietin is easy in hemodialysis patients, it may represent a stressful burden in non-dialysed children and children on peritoneal dialysis in whom it is given subcutaneously. Prolonged half-life and reduction in the total weekly dose can be achieved by injecting erythropoietin subcutaneously. However, this method is associated with real discomfort in young children. The development of the long-acting erythropoietin darbepoietin-alfa, with a long mean terminal half-life of 43 hours, may represent a significant advantage in allowing less frequent dosing [22, 23]. The subcutaneous injection of darbepoietin has been claimed to be more painful than the traditional erythropoietin-beta [24].

Renal osteodystrophy

Phosphate-binders. Hyperphosphataemia is a key factor in the pathogenesis of renal osteodystrophy.
Phosphate binding agents are necessary in many children with chronic renal failure and most children undergoing standard dialysis regimens [25, 26]. Aluminum-based binders carry the risk of aluminum toxicity, leading to encephalopathy, osteomalacia, myopathy and microcystic anaemia. Calcium-based binders may increase the total body calcium load, potentially increasing the risk of cardiovascular and soft tissue calcification. A new compound, *Sevelamer*, is the first phosphate-binder that is calcium-free and metal-free. This agent has been shown to effectively control phosphorus levels in adult patients with renal failure. It also may attenuate coronary and aortic calcifications in adults, although this has not been demonstrated in children. It appears to have beneficial effects on lipid metabolism and inflammation. Preliminary data suggest that sevelamer can also be given safely to children [27]. The risk of inducing chronic metabolic acidosis should not however be overlooked [28].

Calcimimetics. Treatment of secondary hyperparathyroidism with calcium and vitamin D metabolites in patients on dialysis may be complicated by hypercalcaemia and hyperphosphataemia. Calcimimetics target the calcium-sensing receptors (CaSR) and lower parathyroid hormone levels without increasing calcium and phosphorus. Cinacalcet hydrochloride is effective in reducing parathyroid hormone levels in hemodialysed patients with uncontrolled secondary hyperparathyroidism [29]. Experimental evidence suggests that calcimimetic agents may also impede the development of parathyroid gland hyperplasia and increase bone mass [30]. While the effects of calcimimetics on the secretion of parathyroid hormone in children are probably similar to those described in adults, it should be kept in mind that epiphyseal growth plate expresses the CaSR, and that the role of CaSR as a potential modifier of chondrocyte proliferation and differentiation remains uncertain [31].

Transplantation

Chronic allograft nephropathy (CAN) is the leading cause of late graft loss in renal transplantation. It is defined as progressive renal failure associated with hypertension and proteinuria in renal transplant recipients. Histologically, CAN is characterized by afferent arteriolar sclerosis, tubular atrophy, and glomerulosclerosis. The course of CAN is progressive and ultimately leads to graft loss. While the use of calcineurin inhibitors (cyclosporine, tacrolimus) has significantly reduced the rate and severity of acute rejection, and improved graft survival, it has also been associated with the development of histological changes of the renal parenchyma responsible for CAN, with consequent deterioration of GFR and arterial hypertension. Withdrawal or diminished calcineurin-inhibitor therapy may result in rapid improvement of renal function.

Mycophenolate mofetil is an immunosuppressant without nephrotoxicity. When used in combination with steroids and calcineurin inhibitors, MMF has been shown to reduce the rate of acute rejection episodes and improve states of refractory rejection. In recent paediatric studies, MMF improved both short-term and long-term renal function, and reduced blood pressure, probably as a result of concurrent calcineurin-inhibitor reduction [32-34]. A recent meta-analysis in adults has shown that calcineurin-inhibitor withdrawal improves GFR [35]. Steroid and anti-calcineurin-sparing protocols using MMF are now being actively developed [36].

Acute renal failure in the neonates

Asphyxia and respiratory disorders

Theophylline. In neonates, fetal and perinatal hypoxia and asphyxia are the major causes of acute renal failure. The overactivation of intrarenal adenosine seems to play a key role in the pathogenesis of the hypoxemic vasomotor nephropathy (*figure 1*). In experimental studies, theophylline, a non-specific antagonist of adenosine surface cell receptors, prevents the drop in GFR induced by a hypoxemic stress [37]. Recent clinical studies seem to confirm the beneficial effect of theophylline in preventing the renal vasoconstriction induced by hypoxia. Significant improvement in plasma creatinine, creatinine clearance and fluid balance have indeed been demonstrated in asphyxiated neonates [38-40] given prophylactic theophylline (*figure 2*), thus confirming the results described previously by Huet *et al.* [41]. Theophylline has also been beneficial in premature neonates with oliguria secondary to respiratory distress syndrome (RDS) [42]. The rationale for the use of theophylline thus appears promising in oliguric neonates. The safety of adenosine-receptor blockade should however clearly be assessed before recommending the routine use of theophylline in oliguric neonates with respiratory disorders.

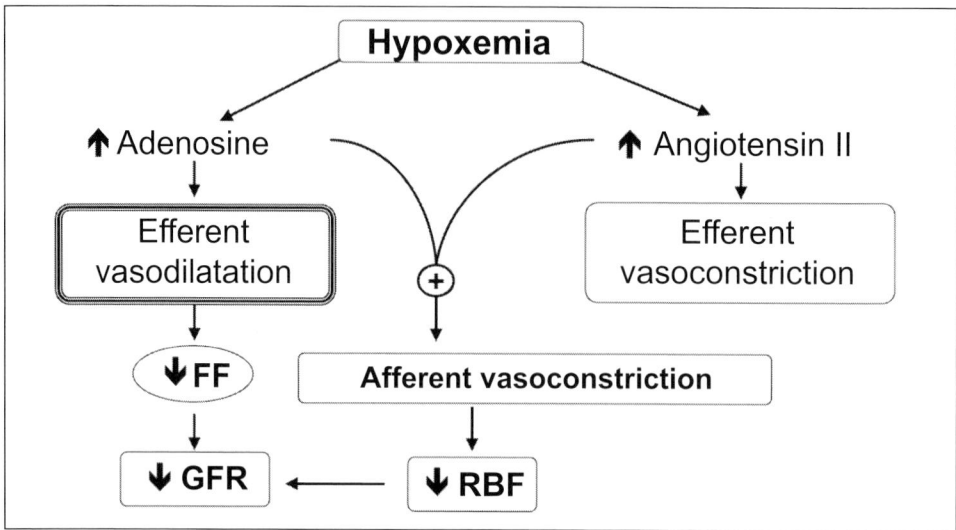

Figure 1. Hypoxemia activates the release of intrarenal adenosine and angiotensin II. While angiotensin II preferentially vasoconstricts the efferent arteriole, adenosine effectively vasodilates it. The decrease in the filtration fraction reflects net efferent vasodilation. The combined net effect of angiotensin II and adenosine is thus afferent vasoconstriction and efferent vasodilation. This results in a decrease in the glomerular pressure, and consequently in GFR.

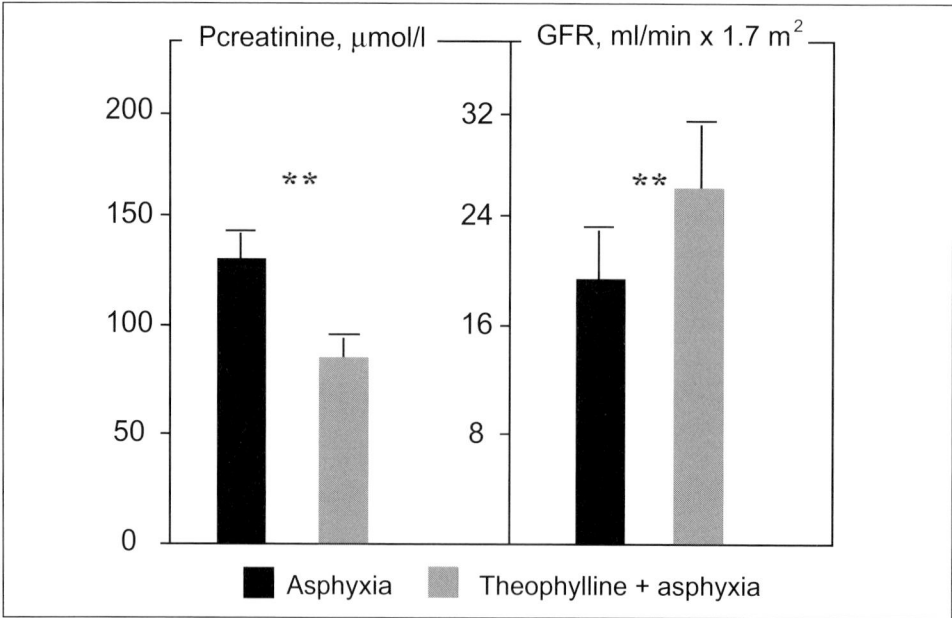

Figure 2. Asphyxiated neonates given prophylactic theophylline have lower plasma creatinine and higher creatinine clearance levels on day 3, as compared to control neonates (Jenik 2000).

Furosemide

Neonates with severe RDS often present with oliguria. The administration of furosemide to these neonates, in the hope of improving renal function, has produced conflicting results. While furosemide usually induces diuresis and a transient improvement in pulmonary function, a critical survey of the literature failed to support the routine use of furosemide in preterm infants with RDS [43]. A recent meta-analysis also concluded that there was not enough evidence to recommend the administration of furosemide in oliguric preterm infants treated with indomethacin for patent ductus arteriosus (PDA) [44]. Clearly, furosemide should not be used to treat oliguric neonates, but primarily neonates with oedematous states and congestive heart failure.

Dopamine

Low-dose dopamine, the so called "renal dose" (0.5-2.5 ug/kg per min) has been widely used in the hope of improving compromised renal function in neonates. While favourable results have initially been described, the great overlap in the response to dopamine and significant inter-individual variability [45, 46] make the beneficial effect of dopamine highly questionable. In addition, detrimental effects following dopamine have been described [47-49].
In adult patients, the results of several randomized controlled trials of low-dose dopamine in critically ill-patients did not show renal sparing; moreover several studies suggest a serious toxic potential of dopamine [50-53].

Vesicoureteric reflux (VUR)

Vesicoureteric reflux is present in approximately 1% of neonates and infants and often resolves spontaneously over the years. The yearly disappearance rate of VUR approximates 13% in mild cases, and 5% in severe (grades IV-V) cases. Bilateral VUR resolves more slowly than unilateral reflux, and more rapidly in boys than in girls [54]. VUR is found in up to 50% of infants with urinary tract infection (UTI) and has been considered as a major risk factor for renal damage. Severe VUR is often familial, different modes of inheritance being involved. Because of the possible risk associated with VUR, two types of preventive measures have been proposed: 1) the surgical or the endoscopic correction of VUR, and 2) prolonged antibiotic prophylaxis.

Well-planned studies have compared the outcome of medical versus surgical treatment in children with severe bilateral VUR and bilateral nephropathy. A 4-year follow-up showed similar results in the functional renal outcome of both medical and surgical treatments [55]. These results did not lend support to the view that the outcome for renal function could be improved by surgical reimplantation of the ureters in children with bilateral nephropathy.

Renal damage can also occur without demonstrable VUR. There is a growing body of evidence indicating that in cases of severe reflux nephropathy, the parenchymal damage is congenital in nature and reflects antenatal dysplasia [56]. In children with exclusively acquired damage due to pyelonephritis, the risk of developing severe nephropathy is probably considerably smaller than previously assumed, at least in conditions when prompt diagnosis and treatment of urinary tract infection is possible. Careful studies by Ismaili *et al.* [56, 57] have provided new insights into the pathogenesis, clinical diagnosis, as well as in the consequences and management of VUR. These observations and relevant conclusions are summarized in an excellent recent review [58].

Investigation of VUR

While micturating cysto-urethrography (MCU) is the method of choice for diagnosing posterior urethral valves and for detecting reflux, its use is associated with significant radiation of the gonadal region and the need for catheterization/puncture of the bladder. The meta-analysis of Gordon *et al.* [59] shows that primary VUR detected by cystography is a weak predictor of renal isotopic DMSA defects, and that the absence of demonstrable VUR by no means rules out such a defect. This study supports the contention that primary VUR is never sufficient on its own, nor is it essential for the development of renal damage in the presence of UTI. In individuals who have been hospitalized with UTI, MCU should not be used as a screening tool to exclude renal defects [59].

MCU is of course mandatory when the presence of posterior urethral valves is suspected. However, its undertaking in other circumstances is controversial, with a tendancy away from its use in all children with renal tract abnormalities or UTI. Some clinicians believe that an MCU does not affect the management because most VURs will resolve spontaneously and there is little evidence to show any benefit from interventions such as antibiotic prophylaxis or surgery. Other authors believe that it is always important to be aware of reflux in order to prevent renal scarring. Unfortunately there is little evidence to support either view, although most would agree that MCU is necessary in the child with dilated ureters or calyceal dilatation.

Surgical and endoscopic correction of reflux

Success in curing VUR with surgical reimplantation is greater than 95% overall. Clearly however, its high success rate by no means justifies this type of surgery in all cases! Reimplantation is indeed a major operation not devoid of risks. Interestingly, pregnant women who have undergone ureteral reimplantation in childhood present apparently with a higher risk of progressive hydronephrosis, UTI, hypertension, renal failure, spontaneous abortion, and premature death [60, 61].

Endoscopic correction of reflux can be effected by injecting tissue-augmenting substances (polytetraflouroethylene, silicon, dextranomer microspheres, collagen) subureterically at the ureterovesical junction. The success rate of endoscopic treatment is considerably lower than that of surgical correction. It is better in low-grades of VUR. A recent meta-analysis of endoscopic therapy revealed resolution of reflux in 79% of ureters with grade I and II, in 72% with grade III and in 65% with grade IV refluxes, following a single injection of the bulking agent [62]. The potential migration of the injected material to other sites as well as extensive granulomatous reactions to the product, are serious causes of concern and may outweigh the possible benefit of endoscopic manoeuvres.

Antibiotic prophylaxis

For many years it has been widely accepted that antibiotic prophylaxis should be considered in all children with VUR. This view has been challenged by a recent multicenter controlled study where antibiotic prophylaxis failed to decrease the rate of recurrent UTI, the type of recurrrence, the rate of subsequent pyelonephritis, and the development of parenchymal scars [63]. The majority of clinicians would treat infants and young children at risk for pyelonephritic scarring (dilated reflux, previous scars, severe obstructive uropathy), children with infections related to nephrolithiasis, and children with voiding disturbances and recurrent UTIs. The use of antibiotic prophylaxis is based on the assumption that uninfected primary reflux does not initiate new renal scars and that most reflux will resolve with time. When prophylaxis is used, it should cover the period at highest risk, that is the first years of life.

Circumcision

Circumcision has been claimed to be effective in preventing UTI in young boys. A meta-analysis of 12 studies assessing the association between UTI and circumcision demonstrates that 111 routine circumcisions would be required to prevent one UTI in normal boys. The ratio is considered better in boys with grade III or more VUR, 4 circumcisions being required to prevent one infection [64]. Incidentally it is interesting to note that three very recent randomised trials have provided firm evidence that the risk of acquiring HIV is halved by male circumcision [65].

Nephron deficit

In 1992, DJ Barker developed his fascinating hypothesis on the fetal and infant origins of adult disease [66]. This hypothesis was based on the observation of an association between birth-weight and the occurrence of cardiovascular diseases at an adult age. Various mechanisms have been proposed to explain the fetal origin of adult renal disease.

Low birth-weight, in particular when associated with intra-uterine growth retardation (IUGR), shows a strong association with the occurrence of adult kidney diseases. Low-birth weight is also associated with a congenital reduction in the number of nephrons [67] (*figure 3*). The deficit in nephrons results in compensatory adaptation of existing nephrons manifested by glomerular hypertrophy and increased single nephron glomerular filtration (hyperfiltration). Chronic hyperfiltration, mediated by activation of the renin-angiotensin-aldosterone system (RAAS) leads to glomerulosclerosis and hypertension, and ultimately to end-stage renal failure [68]. Low birth-weight is usually related to intrauterine growth retardation, secondary to maternal malnutrition or placental insufficiency, or to premature birth. In animal studies, the following factors or agents have been shown to result in a congenital nephron deficit [69]: a low maternal protein diet; maternal vitamin A [70] and iron deficiency; fetal exposure to hyperglycemia, an excess of

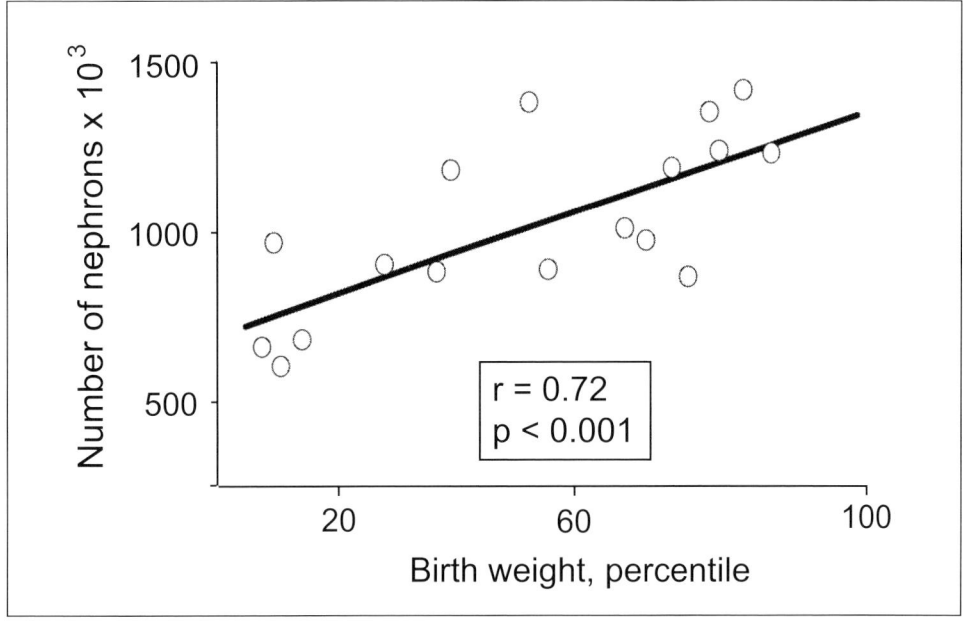

Figure 3. In humans, the number of nephrons correlates positively with birth weight, expressed in percentiles (adapted from C. Merlet-Benichou, *et al.* 1999).

glucocorticoid hormones, beta-lactam antibiotics (ampicillin and amoxicillin) and cyclosporin [71].

In addition to these factors, excessive catch-up growth could well enhance the risk of adult disease. Well-planned recent prospective studies clearly demonstrate that at the age of 19 years, low-birth weight is associated with: 1) an increase in serum creatinine concentration and albuminuria; 2) a decrease GFR in young adults born very preterm; and 3) reduced renal function, the more so in premature neonates born with IUGR [72]. Presently available observations thus suggest that very premature and intrauterine growth-retarded neonates have an increased risk of developing progressive renal failure later in life [73] and that birth-weight should be used as a surrogate marker for future risk of adult disease [74]. Interestingly enough, reduced nephron number observed in Australia aborigines appears to correlate with the susceptibility to chronic kidney disease present in this population [75]. The risks for developing renal failure associated with prematurity and IUGR (*figure 4*) warrants long-term follow-up of all infants born with a low-birth weight. Screening for albuminuria, proteinuria, and hypertension in this group of patients will help in detecting at an early stage those patients who may benefit from active nephroprotection.

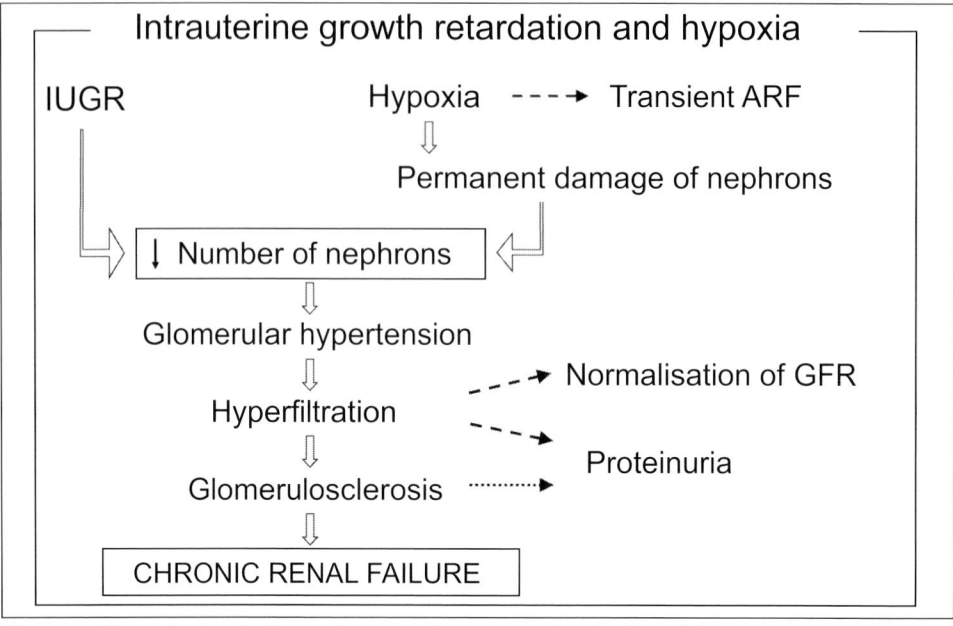

Figure 4. The reduction in the number of nephrons associated with IUGR leads to a compensatory increase in intraglomerular pressure, hyperfiltration, glomerulosclerosis, and ultimately chronic renal failure. Hypoxic stress further decreases the number of functioning nephrons. Proteinuria is often the first sign of glomerulosclerosis.

Nephroprotection

The loss of nephrons, whether acute or chronic, is associated with compensatory hyperfiltration in the remnant nephrons. The RAAS plays a key-role in this phenomenon. By increasing the intra-glomerular pressure, angiotensin II induces single nephron hyperfiltration. Sustained activation of angiotensin II produces systemic and renal side effects: arterial hypertension, mesangial cell proliferation and renal interstitial fibrosis [76]. The renal injury leads to a progressive, relentless deterioration of renal function. Recent clinical trials indicate that blockade of the renin-angiotensin system effectively retards the progression towards end-stage renal failure [77]. A decrease in proteinuria occurs concomitantly [78]. Treatment with angiotensin-converting enzyme inhibitors (ACEI) has been found to be renoprotective in patients with diabetic and non-diabetic chronic renal disease. Treatment with angiotensin II AT1 receptor blockers (ARB) also affords renal protection. Combined treatment with ARBs and ACEIs in non-diabetic renal disease appears more effective in reducing the proteinuria than with ACEIs or ARBs given alone [79, 80]. Neither ACEis nor ARBs completely abrogate the progression of chronic renal disease. This suggests that these agents do not predictably suppress aldosterone, a phenomenon coined as *"aldosterone synthesis escape"*, leaving potentially detrimental effects of aldosterone unabated [81]. Interestingly enough, in recent clinical studies, spironolactone effectively reduced the proteinuria and retarded the progression of renal disease in non-diabetic patients already treated with ACEIs and ARBs [82]. Clinical trials on the effect of ACEIs in retarding the progression of renal disease in children are under way. A short-term (6 months) study with ramipril showed that this agent effectively and safely improved the proteinuria and hypertension in children with renal disease [83]. In a more recent 6 month-study in 10 proteinuric children with renal disease, the combination of ACEIs and ARBs significantly reduced the proteinuria, as compared with baseline or either drug alone. In addition, echocardiographic examination of these children provided evidence of reduced left ventricular hypertrophy [84]. Clinical long-term trials on the effect of ACEIs or ARBs on the progression of chronic renal disease in children are not yet available. Short-term observations give real hope that the progression of chronic renal diseases in children will be abated by the early use of AEIs and/or ARBs.

References

1. Gubler MC. Congenital and infantile nephrotic syndromes. In: Guignard JP, GouyonJB, Simeoni U, eds. *Développement rénal et programmation des maladies cardiovasculaires*. Paris: Elsevier, 2005: 83-92.
2. Putaala H, Soininen R, Kilpeläinen P, *et al*. The murin nephrin gene is specifically expressed in kidney, brain and pancreas: inactivation of the gene leads to massive proteinuria and neonatal death. *Hum Mol Genet* 2001; 10: 1-8.
3. Heidet L, Bongers EM, Sich M, *et al*. *In vivo* expression of putative *LMX1B* targets in nail-patella syndrome kidneys. *Am J Pathol* 2003; 163: 145-55.
4. Antignac C, Arduy C, Beckmann JS, *et al*. A gene for familiar juvenile nephronophtisis maps to chromosome 2p. *Nat Genet* 1993; 3: 342-5.
5. Hildebrandt F, Singh-Sawhney I, Schnieders B, *et al*. Mapping of a gene for familial juvenile nephronophtisis: refining the map and defining flanking markers on chromosome 2. *Am J Hum Genet* 1993; 53: 1256-61.
6. Saunier S, Salsman R, Antignac C. Nephronophtisis. *Curr Op Genet Dev* 2005; 15: 324-31.
7. Coulter MB, Lian Q. Consequences of misense mutations for dimerization and turnover of alanine: glyoxylate aminotransferase: study of a spectrum of mutations. *Mol Genet Metab* 2006: 89: 345-55.
8. Cochat P, Liutkus A. Primary hyperoxaluria type 1: still challenging. *Pediatr Nephrol* 2006; 8: 1075-81.
9. Webster KE, Ferree PM, Holmes RP, Cramer SD. Identification of missense, nonsense, and delation mutations in the GRHPR gene in patients with primary hyperoxaluria type II (PH2). *Hum Genet* 2000; 107: 176-85.
10. Zelikovic I. Molecular pathophysiology of tubular transport disorders. *Pediatr Nephrol* 2001; 16: 919-25.
11. Filler G, Bökenkamp A, Hofmann W, *et al*. Cystatin C as a marker of GFR: history, indications, and future research. *Clin Biochem* 2005; 38: 1-8.
12. Grubb A, Nyman U, Björk J, *et al*. Simple Cystatin C-based prediction equations for glomerular filtration rate compared with the modification of diet in renal disease prediction equation for adults and the Schwartz and the Counahan-Barratt prediction equations for children. *Clin Chem* 2005; 51: 1420-31.
13. Knight EL, Verhave JC, Spiegelman D, *et al*. Factors influencing serum systatin C levels other than renal function and the impact on renal function measurement. *Kidney Int* 2004; 65: 1416-21.

14. Risch L, Herklotz R, Blumberg A, Huber AR. Effects of glucocorticoid immunosuppression on serum Cystatin C concentrations in renal transplant patients. *Clin Chem* 2001; 47: 2055-9.
15. Mendiluce A, Bustamante J, Martin D, et al. Cystatin C as a marker of renal function in kidney transplant patients. *Transplant Proc* 2005; 37: 3844-7.
16. Martini S, Prevot A, Mosig D, Guignard JP. Glomerular filtration rate: measure creatinine and height rather that cystatin C! *Acta Paediatr* 2003; 92: 1052-7.
17. Bagga A, Hari P, Moudgil A, Jordan SC. Mycophenolate mofetil and prednisolone therapy in children with steroid-dependent nephrotic syndrome. *Am J Kidney Dis* 2003; 42: 1114-20.
18. Ulinski T, Dubourg L, Said MH, et al. Switch from cyclosporine A to mycophenolate mofetil in nephrotic children. *Pediatr Nephrol* 2005; 20: 482-5.
19. Fujinaga S, Ohtomo Y, Umino D, et al. A prospective study on the use of mycophenolate mofetil in children with cyclosporin-dependent nephrotic syndrome. *Pediatr Nephrol* 2007; 22: 71-6.
20. Novak I, Frank R, Vento S, et al. Efficacy of mycophenolate mofetil in pediatric patients with steroid-dependent nephrotic syndrome. *Pediatr Nephrol* 2005; 20: 1265-8.
21. Ulinski T, Carlier-Legris A, Schlecht D, et al. Triamcinolone acetonide: a new management of noncompliance in nephrotic children. *Pediatr Nephrol* 2005; 20: 759-62.
22. Lerner G, Kale AS, Warady BA, Jabs K, et al. Pharmacokinetics of darbepoetin alfa in pediatric patients with chronic kidney disease. *Pediatr Nephrol* 2002; 17: 933-7.
23. De Palo T, Giordano M, Palumbo F, et al. Clinical experience with darbepoietin alfa (NESP) in children undergoing hemodialysis. *Pediatr Nephrol* 2004; 19: 337-40.
24. Schmitt CP, Nau B, Brummer C, et al. Increased injection pain with darbepoetin-alfa compared to epoetin-beta in paediatric dialysis patients. *Nephrol Dial Transplant* 2006; 21: 3520-4.
25. Salusky IB. A new area in phosphate binder therapy: What are the options? *Kidney Int* 2006; 70: S10-5.
26. Waller S, Ridout D, Cantor T, Rees L. Parathyroid hormone and growth in children with chronic renal failure. *Kidney Int* 2005; 67: 2338-45.
27. Querfeld U. The therapeutic potential of novel phosphate binders. *Pediatr Nephrol* 2005; 20: 389-92.
28. Pieper AK, Haffner D, Hoppe B, et al. A randomized crossover trial comparing sevelamer with calcium acetate in children with CKD. *Am J Kidney Dis* 2006; 47: 625-35.
29. Block GA, Martin KJ, de Francisco AL, et al. Cinacalcet for secondary hyperparathyroidism in patients receiving hemodialysis. *N Engl J Med* 2004; 350: 1516-25.
30. Goodman WG. Calcimimetics: a remedy for all problems of excess parathyroid hormone activity in chronic kidney disease. *Curr Opin Nephrol Hypertens* 2005; 14: 355-60.
31. Goodman WG. Calcimimetic agents for the treatment of secondary hyperparathyroidism. *Semin Nephrol* 2004; 24: 460-3.
32. Pape L, Mengel M, Offner G, et al. Renal arterial resistance index and computorized quantification of fibrosis as a combined predictive tool in chronic allograft nephropathy? *Pediatr Transplant* 2004; 8: 565-70.
33. Kerecuk L, Taylor J, Clark G. Chronic allograft nephropathy and mycophenolate mofetil introduction in paediatric renal recipients. *Pediatr Nephrol* 2005; 20: 1630-5.
34. Otukesh H, Sharifian M, Basiri A, et al. Mycophenolate mofetil in pediatric renal transplantation. *Transplant Proc* 2005; 37: 3012-5.
35. Mulay AV, Hussain N, Fergusson D, Knoll GA. Calcineurin inhibitor withdrawal from sirolimus-based therapy in kidney transplantation: a systematic review of randomized trials. *Am J Transplant* 2005; 5: 1748-56.
36. Land W, Vincenti F. Toxicity-sparing protocols using mycophenolate mofetil in renal transplantation. *Transplantation* 2005; 80: S221-34.
37. Gouyon JB, Guignard JP. Theophylline prevents the hypoxemia-induced renal hemodynamic changes in rabbits. *Kidney Int* 1988; 33: 1078-83.
38. Jenik AG, Ceriani Cernadas JM, Gorenstein A, et al. A randomized, double-blind, placebo-controlled trial of the effects of prophylactic theophylline on renal function in term neonates with perinatal asphyxia. *Pediatrics* 2000; 105: e45.

39. Bakr AF. Prophylactic theophylline to prevent renal dysfunction in newborns exposed to perinatal asphyxia – a study in a developing country. *Pediatr Nephrol* 2005; 20: 1249-52.
40. Bhat M, Shah ZA, MakhdoomiMS, Mufti MH. Theophylline for renal function in term neonates with perinatal asphyxia: a randomized, placebo-controlled trial. *J Pediatr* 2006; 14: 180-4.
41. Huet F, Semama D, Grimaldi M, *et al*. Effects of theophylline on renal insufficiency in neonates with respiratory distress syndrome. *Intensive Care Med* 1995; 21: 511-4.
42. Cattarelli D, Spandrio M, Gasparoni A, *et al*. A randomized, double-blind, placebo-controlled trial of the effect of theophylline in prevention of vasomotor nephropathy in very preterm neonates with respiratory distress syndrome. *Arch Dis Child Fetal Neonatal Ed* 2006; 91: F80-4.
43. Brion LP, Soll RF. Diuretics for respiratory distress syndrome in preterm infants. *Cochrane Database Syst Rev* 2001; 2: CD001454.
44. Barrington K, Brion LP. Dopamine versus no treatment to prevent renal dysfunction in indomethacin-treated preterm newborn infants. *Cochrane Database Syst Rev* 2002; (3): CD003213.
45. Seri I, Abbasi S, Wood DC, Gerdes JS. Regional hamodynamic effects of dopamine in the indomethacin-treated preterm infant. *J Perinatol* 2002; 22: 300-5.
46. Lynch SK, Lemley KV, Polak MJ. The effects of dopamine on glomerular filtration rate in normotensive, oliguric premature neonates. *Pediatr Nephrol* 2003; 18: 649-52.
47. Holmes CL, Walley KR. Bad medicine: Low-dose dopamine in the ICU. *Chest* 2003; 124: 1266-75.
48. Rice BA, Tanski MC. The case against renal dose dopamine in the pediatric intensive care unit. *AACN Clin Issues* 2005; 16: 246-51.
49. Lauschke A, Teichgraber UK, Frei U, Eckardt KU. "Low-dose" dopamine worsens renal perfusion in patients with acute renal failure. *Kidney Int* 2006; 69: 1669-74.
50. Thompson BI, Cockrill BA. Renal-dose dopamine: A siren song. *Lancet* 1994; 344: 7-8.
51. Kellum JA, Decker JM. Use of dopamine in acute renal failure: a meat-analysis. *Crit Care Med* 2001; 29: 1526-31.
52. Padmanabhan R. Renal dose dopamine: the myth and the truth. *J Assoc Physicians India* 2002; 50: 571-5.
53. Friederich JO, Adhikari N, Herridge MS, Beyene J. Meta-analysis: low-dose dopamine increases urine output but does not prevent renal dysfunction or death. *Ann Intern Med* 2005; 142: 510-24.
54. Schwab CW, Wu HY, Selman H, *et al*. Spontaneous resolution of vesicoureteral reflux: a 15-year perspective. *J Urol* 2002; 168: 2594-9.
55. Smellie JM, Barratt TM, Chantler C, *et al*. Medical versus surgical treatment in children with severe bilateral vesicouretic reflux and bilateral nephropathy: a randomised trial. *Lancet* 2001; 357: 1329-33.
56. Ismaili K, Avni FB, Wissing KM, Hall M. Long-term clinical outcome of infants with mild and moderate fetal pyeloectasis: validation of neonatal ultrasound as a screening tool to detect significant nephro-uropathies. *J Pediatr* 2004; 16: 4-7.
57. Ismaili K, Hall M, Piepsz A, *et al*. Primary vesicoureteral reflux detected among neonates with a history of fetal pelvis dilatation: A prospective clinical and imaging study. *J Pediatr* 2006; 148: 222-7.
58. Ismaili K, Avni FE, Piepsz A, *et al*. Vesicoureteric reflux in children. *EAU-EBU Update Series* 2006; 4: 129-40.
59. Gordon I, Barkovics M, Pindoria S, *et al*. Primary vesicouretic relux as a predictor of renal damage in children hospitalized with urinary tract infection: A systematic review and meta-analysis. *J Am Soc Nephrol* 2003; 14: 739-44.
60. Bukowski TP, Betros GG, Aquilina JW, Perlmutter AD. Urinary tract infections and pregnancy in women who underwent antireflux surgery in childhood. *J Urol* 1998; 159: 1286-9.
61. Mor Y, Leibovitch I, Friedmans A, *et al*. Late post-reimplantation ureteral obstruction during pregnancy: a transient phenomenon? *J Urol* 2003; 170: 845-8.

62. Elder JS, Peters CA, Arant BS, et al. Pediatric Vesicoureteral Reflux Guidelines Panel summary report on the management of primary vesicoureteral reflux in children. *J Urol* 1997; 157: 1846-51.
63. Garin EH, Olavarria F, Garcia Nieto V, et al. Clinical significance of primary vesicoureteral reflux and urinary antibiotic prophylaxix after acute pyelonephritis: a multicenter, randomized, controlled study. *Pediatrics* 2006; 117: 626-32.
64. Singh-Grewal D, Macdessi J, Craig J. Circumcision for the prevention of urinary tract infection in boys: a systematic review of randomized trials and obstruction studies. *Arch Dis Child* 2005; 90: 853-8.
65. Editorial comment. Male circumcision to cut HIV risk in the general population. Lancet 2007; 369: 617-9.
66. Barker DJ. Fetal and Infant Origins of Adult Disease. London: BMJ Publisher.1992.
67. Merlet-Bénichou C, Gilbert T, Vilar J, et al. Nephron number: Variability is the rule. Causes and consequences. *Lab Invest* 1999; 79: 515-27.
68. Zandi-Nejad K, Luyckx VA, Brenner BM. Adult hypertension and kidney disease: The role of fetal programming. *Hypertension* 2006; 47: 502-8.
69. Lelièvre-Pegorier M, Merlet-Bénichou C. The number of nephrons in the mammalian kidney: environmental influences play a determining role. *Exp Nephrol* 2000; 8: 63-5.
70. Gilbert T, Merlet-Benichou C. Retinoids and nephron mass control. *Pediatr Nephrol* 2000; 14: 1137-44.
71. Tendron-Franzin A, Gouyon JB, Guignard JP, et al. Long-term effects of *in utero* exposure to cyclosporin A on renal function in the rabbit. *J Am Nephrol Assoc* 2004; 15: 2687-93.
72. Keijzer-Veen MG, Schrevel M, Finken MJ, et al. Microalbuminuria and lower filtration rate at young adult age in subjects born very prematurely and after intrauterine growth retardation. *J Am Soc Nephrol* 2005; 16: 2762-8.
73. Rodriguez-Soriano J, Aguirre M, Oliveros R, Vallo A. Long-term renal follow-up of extremely low birth weight infants. *Pediatr Nephrol* 2005; 20: 579-84.
74. Luyckx VA, Brenner BM. Low birth weight, nephron number, and kidney disease. *Kidney Int* 2005; 97: S68-77.
75. Hoy WE, Hughson MD, Singh GR, et al. Reduced nephron number and glomerulomegaly in Australian Aborigines: a group at high risk for renal disease and hypertension. *Kidney Int* 2006; 70: 104-10.
76. Ma LJ, Fogo AB. Role of angiotensin II in glomerular injury. *Semin Nephrol* 2001; 21: 544-53.
77. Taal MW, Brenner BM. Renoprotective benefits of RAS inhibition: From ACEI to angiotensin II antagonists. *Kidney Int* 2000; 57: 1803-17.
78. Zandi-Nejad K, Eddy AA, Glassock RJ, Brener BM. Why is proteinuria an ominous biomarker of progressive kidney disease. *Kidney Int* 2004; 92: S76-89.
79. Nakao N, Yoshimura H, Morita M, et al. Combination treatment of angiotensin-II receptor blocker and angiotensin-converting-enzyme inhibitor in non-diabetic renal disease (COOPERATE): a randomised controlled trial. *Lancet* 2003; 361: 117-24.
80. Zandi-Nejad K, Brenner BM. Strategies to retard the progression of chronic kidney disease. *Med Clin North Am* 2005; 89: 489-509.
81. Aldigier JC, Kanjanbuch T, Ma LJ, et al. Remission of existing glomerulosclerosis by inhibition of aldosterone. *J Am Soc Nephrol* 2005; 16: 3306-14.
82. Bianchi S, Bigazzi R, Campese VM. Long-term effects of spironolactone on proteinuria and kidney function in patients with chronic kidney disease. *Kidney Int* 2006; 70: 2116-23.
83. Seeman T, Dusek J, Vondrak K, Flögelova, Geier P, Janka J. Ramipril in the treatment of hypertension and protenuria in children with chronic kidney diseases. *Am J Hypertens* 2004; 17: 415-20.
84. Lubrano R, Soscia F, Elli M, et al. Renal and cardiovascular effects of angiotensin-converting enzyme inhibitor plus angiotensin II receptor antagonist therapy in children with proteinuria. *Pediatrics* 2006; 118: e822-8.

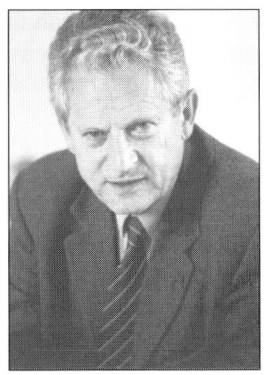

Recent Progress in Child Psychiatry

Philippe JEAMMET

Head of the Department of Psychiatry,
Institut Mutualiste Montsouris, Paris, France

The evolution of knowledge in child psychiatry may seem slower and less spectacular than in other fields of child and adolescent pathology. It is not, however, less profound. We will illustrate that point through three fields of research. Recent developments in child psychiatry are primarily due to findings in neuroscience, genetics and neuroimaging. It should be noted that these findings are inscribed in the development of the personality and its relational context, rendering comprehension particularly complex.

Towards an integrative perspective in the etiopathogenic understanding of psychiatric problems

The past twenty years have witnessed a radical epistemological change. Specifically, a developmental perspective for understanding and considering questions related to

The concept of therapeutic alliance has been considered in adults since the 1970s and was extended into the practice of child psychiatry in the 1980s because of the developments of psychiatry of the baby, psychiatry of the adolescent and peri-natal psychiatry. This development is in part pragmatic: if we wish to reach out to children and keep them in care, it is necessary that their parents find treatment acceptable. It is also related to the increasingly systemic understanding of problems in child psychiatry. We can not work without a child's parents. We can not put the child in a position where he might experience conflicting loyalties. Parents must be partners in care.

Scientific advances no longer allow us to consider parents completely responsible for their child's psychological problems, as many did before 1980. The revolutions in the understandings of autism and transgenerational issues are paradigms of this change. Fraiberg was a pioneer in this field [9].

The revolution of attachment theory

This theory, developed by Bowlby, then elaborated by Ainsworth in the 1970s has been since the 1990s a revolutionary source in the understanding of child development [10]. Today, attachment theory has a role that could be considered analogous to that of psychoanalysis at the beginning of the 20th century.

Based on observations of the reaction of a child to separation, Bowlby reflected upon the nature of mother-child relationships. Theories of "secondary drives" which were elaborated from psychoanalysis or from learning theory were prevalent in his work in the beginning of the 1950s. These theories describe the mother-child relationship as a consequence of maternal gratifications, the most important of which was feeding. In these conceptions, the only primary needs were those of the body.
The work of Lorenz on painting, which led many to question these theories, led Bowlby to the hypothesis that there existed primary attachment behaviour capable of linking the child to his mother. For Bowlby, the proclivity to establish strong affective links with particular people is one of the fundamental components of human nature.

He progressively elaborated his cybernetic theory of attachment behaviour which attempts to explain the constitution of all affective links, not only those between mother and child but also those between adults.

Although this theoretical elaboration was facilitated by Bowlby's initial training, psychoanalysis, and by ethology, the theory is greatly eclectic and also involves principals related to cybernetic theory of regulation or systems theory, neurophysiology, developmental psychology and cognitive psychology.

Ethology presented the idea that social behaviour has an instinctive dimension and that relationships can be observed experimentally. Psychoanalytic theory (object relations) presents the notion of an internal world including representations of the self, of others and relationships between the two, with these representations potentially deformed by immaturity or fantasies.

According to attachment theory, the affective relationship between the child and his mother is the product of attachment behaviour. The system of attachment behaviour regroups and organizes the totality of signal and approach behaviours with the result of obtaining or maintaining a proximity in relation to another, preferred person, most often the mother.

This system develops from the first months of life. Starting from birth, the baby is capable of social interaction and shows pleasure in this. During the first few weeks, the baby already manifests a great number of constitutive reactions which will become attachment behaviour. However, this behaviour can not really be organized in a system in regards to a discriminate figure until the child has the cognitive ability to remember his mother when she is not present, an ability which develops during the second semester of life. It is therefore around nine months that an organized system is in place and it reaches a typical form during the second year. It is activated by the departure of the mother or any alarming situation and deactivates when the child can see, hear or touch his mother. After three years of age, the activation of this behavioural system is less frequent and its deactivation becomes possible through a growing number of conditions, sometimes only symbolic.

Therefore, progressively, more than the effective presence of the attachment figure, representation models of this figure's availability will play the principal role.

In light of these modifications, the attachment behaviour and the links to which they lead will persist throughout the lifetime, although the figures towards which they are directed may change.

The experiences with attachment figures in early childhood until adolescence determine adult attachment behaviour. This is an essential point of Bowlby's theory, who considered that the attachment schema developed by an individual during childhood was modeled by the attitude of his parents and then persists, becoming a quality specific to that individual, which will then affect his new relationships with others.

Two general types of attachment were described:
– "Confidant" or "Secure" attachment, in which contact with the attachment figure is without ambivalence, facilitating separations;

- "Insecure" attachment, subdivided into:
    - "Insecure-avoidant" attachment: there exists an avoidance of the attachment figure; contact is not sought out but is not refused either.
    - "Insecure-ambivalent" attachment: the contact is sought out, but it seems to be avoided at the same time. The child might protest when picked up by his mother but also protest when put down. For this type of attachment, we speak of anxious attachment.
    - "Insecure-disorganized/disoriented" attachment: Apprehension, confusion, even depression are seen in the child.

To account for the persistence of an attachment schema in an individual, Bowlby uses the concept of internal operating models of one's self and of one's parents. These mental models are constructed during the first years on the basis of real experiences. These experiences reflect the parents and the child himself as a function of the image that the parents have of the child. Mental models persist even after circumstances have been modified.

Therefore, attachment behaviour has its own, distinct dynamic with an equal biological signification to eating behaviour or sexual behaviour. The links to which it leads exist on their own, in interaction with those determined by feeding and sexuality. They have in and of themselves a vital function.

These homeostatic behaviour systems permanently maintain the real or symbolic distance from the attachment figure within certain limits. Any differences between the initial instructions and the execution in process modify the behaviour as a result.

Many intense emotions are the outcome of this attachment relationship. Its maintenance and renewal bring about joy and feelings of security. Its break-down can lead to anxiety if temporary or grief if definitive.

According to Bowlby, pathology results from a deviant evolution of attachment behaviour, which in most cases is at the origin of a too frequent activation of this behaviour, leading to anxious attachment. The strongest forms of attachment behaviour are provoked by the threat of loss (the equivalent is observed in the child during the protestation phase). In certain cases, these threats arise frequently, leading to anxiety disorders like school phobia or agoraphobia. The equivalent of the despair phase could also more easily be prolonged in certain individuals confronted by situations of loss. Because of deviations during development, these individuals with irregular attachment behaviour might develop depression.

The modalities of attachment links created in early childhood, as they have been described, are stable and may be altered only by exceptional circumstances (deaths, traumas, meetings, psychotherapy).

At the end of adolescence, the attachment system that until this point has been marked by the asymmetry of relationships becomes symmetric between individuals having reached the same stage of psychological development. Attachment relationships become more reciprocal.

At the heart of these adult relationships, important differences exist between friendly relationships represented by auxiliary attachment figures and the love relationship, which represents after around two or three years, the principal attachment figure.

In most cases, therefore, the sexual partner plays the role of the principal attachment figure in adulthood and takes the place held by the parents during childhood.

More than a global theory of psychological functioning, attachment theory represents a conceptual framework of relationships, and more specifically of aspects of relationships related to security needs. It is, in its essence, a spatial theory: when I am near to this person to whom I am attached, I feel good; when I am far I feel anxious or sad. Attachment is transmitted through sight, sound, and touch, which calm and create the feeling of security that allows the individual to move away and explore.

Towards continuity between psychiatric difficulties in childhood and pathology in adulthood

The development of genetic studies and neurobiology argue in favour of a continuity of psychiatric problems, particularly mood disorders and schizophrenic disorders. The issue has progressively changed from recognition of problems in childhood to the specific mode of expression. The possibility of potential signs of these pathologies in childhood has been raised in the following way: should we speak of childhood disorders or of disorders beginning in childhood? The major problem today is in the possibility of making valid and recognized criteria of the disorder operational. Therefore the identification of a disorder in a child implies the differentiation of this entity from usual experiences related to development and to separate these problems from other pathologies in this age group.

Mood disorders

Major depressive disorder (MDD) is a familial recurrent illness that significantly interferes with a child's normal emotional and cognitive development. MDD is associated with increased risk for suicidal behaviour and suicide attempts, development of other psychiatric disorders (e.g., substance abuse), and work functioning. Child and adolescent onset MDD increases the risk for depressive recurrences and psychosocial difficulties during adulthood [11-13]. The prevalence of MDD in children and adolescents is approximately 2% and 6%, respectively. The most recent research suggests that individuals born more recently are at a greater risk for developing mood disorders, and that these disorders are manifesting at a younger age.

Up to 50% of adults with MDD report that their depression began during childhood. Clinical and community studies have consistently found that adolescent onset MDD is a strong risk factor for adult MDD and is associated with high psychiatric morbidity, personality difficulties, work problems, poor academic performance and potential mortality due to suicide in the young adult years [13-17].

Family factors that influence the course of the disorder may be genetic or nongenetic. Twin and adoption studies show clear evidence of genetic factors' influences on age of onset and recurrence. Family environmental factors, such as exposure to parental depression (e.g., modeling parent's coping styles with stress, poor parental skills or inability to perform parental duties, living with a parent who is frequently irritable, economic difficulties due to parent's inability to work) all may increase the risk for depression [18-20]. Also, factors such as exposure to negative events (e.g., losses, sexual abuse, ongoing conflict) may trigger and perpetuate the depression in certain individuals.

Longitudinal studies in depressed children and adolescents have shown that at follow-up, 5% to 30% of youths with depression will develop mania or hypomania.

Family history for mood disorder, in particular recurrent types in first-degree relatives and child's prior history of mood disorders are risk factors for the onset, duration and recurrence of MDD.

Because MDD is a condition that is prone to relapse and recurrence, it is important that treatment be of sufficient duration to avoid relapse. Studies of short-term treatment have documented the high risk of relapse after discontinuation of psychotherapy or anti-depressant treatment [21]. Both naturalistic and controlled studies of continuation treatment have shown superiority with regard to prevention of relapse, compared to acute treatment alone.

Schizophrenic disorders

Diagnostic criteria is still a subject of research [22]. Difficulties and divergences amongst different authors are even more pronounced concerning the possible forewarning signs of a psychotic evolution.

There is a broadly defined group of children described as having borderline disorder who have noted difficulties with poor reality testing, tumultuous relationships, behavioural and affective dysregulation, and fluctuation between neurotic and psychotic-like states. The overlap in presenting symptoms can make it particularly difficult to differentiate these children from those with schizophrenia. Youth with conduct and other non psychotic emotional disorders may report psychotic-like symptoms, and thus be improperly diagnosed as having a primary psychotic disorder [23].

The presence of hallucinations consisting *"of a voice keeping up a running commentary on the person's behaviour or thoughts, or two or more voices conversing with each other"* (DSM IV) (in other words the classical mental automatisms, de Clérambault), as well as the presence of negative symptoms, remain the best diagnosis.

Among the symptoms, ahedonia and problems of volition are those which have the greatest predictive value and are the most stable. They may reflect a vulnerability which is common to the entire range of schizophrenia, and thus explain the later development of other symptoms even though causality may be different.

Ahedonia is all the more important in that it has always been one of the most specific and troublesome processes of schizophrenia, along with dissociation. It is also interesting to note that this symptom links biological factors, which are becoming more well known, to psychological and developmental factors interacting with the environment.

Are there schizophrenic prodromes? Yung and Mc Gorry [24] pertinently raised the question: *"The initial prodrome in psychosis may be thought of in two ways: first, as the earliest, pre-psychotic form of a psychotic disorder, that is, an attenuated form of psychosis or « emergent psychosis »; second, it may be seen as a syndrome which confers a heightened vulnerability to becoming psychotic, but psychosis is not inevitable. That is, it is a risk factor for psychosis".*

To once again quote Yung and Mc Gorry: *"One important underlying conceptual consideration is whether psychotic symptoms represent qualitatively different phenomena from normal mental experiences or occur on a continuum with normal experiences, representing quantitative deviations only"*. *"A further possibility is that psychotic symptoms represent quantitative differences at onset but at a later point undergo a qualitative change etc."*

And again from Yung and Mc Gorry: *"Like physical systemic disorders, mental disorders probably require environmental stress and an underlying susceptibility. Claridge has suggested that as both of these factors are continuous variables then manifestations of disorder occur on a dimension also, from mild or incomplete through severe. Claridge concludes that a continuity view of psychotic behaviour becomes not just feasible but the most probable explanation of currently available evidence and speculates that there may be a point in the course of the disorder when a qualitative change occurs, as happens in hypertensive disease. The timing and clinical indicators of this point beyond which psychosis will invariably occur are not yet known."*

We completely agree with the way Yung and Mc Gorry envisage these different questions: the meaning of prodromes, the attenuated forms of the disturbance or vulnerability factors, a continuum normal/pathological versus a rupture, a spectrum of susceptibility. However the underlying fundamental question concerning the nature of the pathology as well as that of the vulnerability factors remains unanswered.
Conceptually, schizophrenia is a group of disorders with different clinical profiles and evolutions. Psychological, pharmacological, genetic and neuro-developmental studies have lead to different pathogenetic hypotheses. No one factor is entirely responsible, nor can any one factor be formally eliminated. Schizophrenia is a multi-factorial disorder. The current tendency is to describe a schizophrenic "vulnerability", with a clinical and evolutionary image which depends concurrently on environmental conditions, and on the therapeutic modalities set up to handle these patients.

The place of a developmental perspective in child and adolescent psychiatry

The developmental perspective enlarges the debate because it includes organic data but does not exclude other data. Vulnerability factors, such as self-protection, are also contingent on the nature of the ties that the child had to his surroundings and the quality of his internalizations depending on which, attachments will be either secure or insecure. These ties are also the basis for solid self-esteem and narcissism and a strong self. If the ego is weak it will be more dependent on the fortuity of external relationships. Quantitative changes may, at a given time, lead to a qualitative rupture of the patient's relation to himself, to his self-image or to others.
This dependency can be described as a defensive use of sensory-motor reality to counter-invest an absent or threatening psychic reality. In this perspective, dependency is potentially, if not constantly, present in mental functioning. There is always an interplay between cathexis and counter-cathexis: between internal psychic real-

ity and the external reality of the sensory-motor world. However, the problem arises when dependency becomes a prevalent and permanent mode of functioning, to the detriment of other possibilities. It is a modality which can have bearings on different psychic structures and organizations. Dependency can appear or disappear in function of varying internal and environmental conjunctures, to which, by definition, it is extremely sensitive. Those who become dependent are those who use external reality in a restricting and dominant way; that is to say, those who use the sensory-motor world to counter-invest an inner reality on which they cannot rely, because it does not purvey sufficient security, without sufficient security, relative freedom is not possible. When inner reality provides sufficiently security, it offers a possibility of regression in cases of conflict or difficulty. This regression is not synonymous with disorganization. For a variety of reasons, the inner reality of dependent patients does not have a sufficiently secure foundation.

This dependency on the external world is especially prevalent in potentially psychotic patients whose childhood equilibrium relied largely on external reality and an idealized relationship of dependency on one or several significant others, as a way to counter-invest inner reality. A sudden and brutal questioning of relational distances to these supportive objects brings the patient to realize his dependency, and threatens his narcissistic equilibrium. The reaction may be either excessive distancing or excessive merging.
Furthermore, the emergence of excessive stimuli be they internal or external, which overwhelm the ego's psychic resources, is susceptible to create a traumatic situation by perturbing the differentiation between inside an outside, or between the different intra-psychic functional structures.

Inner bearings vacillate; representations are a source of agitation rather than organization. The only way the ego can protect itself from being submerged is by clinging to perceptual reality. Perceptual reality maintains a minimal differentiation between internal and external, between self and other, except when this reality is itself submerged by hallucinatory or delirious projections. Using perception and motor activity to counter-invest an anxiety-ridden and disorganizing inner reality, is similar to the way a sleeping person, overwhelmed by a nightmare, wakes up and comes back to reality by cutting himself off from his inner world, thanks to the perceptual reality of his familiar surroundings.
The entire relationship to pleasure crumbles. The potentially dependent patient experiences his desire towards others as an intolerable dependency. He feels diminished and threatened by this desire, which he experiences as a need that makes him feel dangerously passive. His desire for others become invasive, and others become a consuming force. This desire is no longer experienced as potentially pleasant, but as another's ascendancy over him. Here we are close to the syndrome of influence, which the patient tries to ward off by acting out. He feels threatened in his personal identity. He is overwhelmed by emotional turmoil and by the intensity of invasive agitation with an inevitable sexual connotation. This excessive turmoil leads to a

situation of non-differentiation: loss of partially acquired differences between internal and external, between the patient and his relationships, and between the different instances of his own psychic apparatus. He is possessed, inhabited by emotional turmoil and by the other that is the cause of this turmoil. The only solution is to expulse the disorganizing agitation onto an outside element over which the patient will try to gain ascendancy and to exercise the omnipotent control which he is incapable of having over his internal agitation. To a different degree, depending on various psychic organizations, everything that comes into contact with these patients is perceived as something imposed on them by someone else. The other is no longer perceived as the object of their own desire but rather as a turmoil-provoking object whose origin is external. The object invades them through affect. It manipulates and takes possession of them, influences them, and in short, strips them of their free-will. Desire enters the patient like a Trojan horse sent by the object.
This is why we feel that the equilibrium between internal resources and the recourse to the external sensory-motor world is so vitally important.

Because of this internal insecurity, narcissistic equilibrium is largely supported by relationships to external objects which are used to counterbalance an internal reality that threatens the patient with disorganization. Internal resources always need external support. However, when a patient is completely tributary to an external presence in order to maintain his internal equilibrium, this presence, especially when it is parental, risks becoming overly sexualized and conflictual at adolescence. It is this type of relationship that adolescence specifically subverts and attempts to demolish. These external objects become sexualized and are no longer idealized. Thus they no longer fulfill their role of providing narcissistic support. At the same time, the adolescent is in need of reinforcing his newfound autonomy, completing his identifications and consolidating his internal acquisitions. This makes him even more dependent on the external object and exacerbates and updates the antagonism between the need for the object and the need for autonomy.

All throughout this period there exists what we will call a common groundwork, which makes this age a critical period, with specific risks. In adolescence and early post-adolescence, we can see, what seem to be childhood vulnerabilities, give way to pathogenic behaviours around which the patient may reorganize his personality and become fixated in repetitious replay, which then may be qualified as pathological. What is not only pathogenic but actually pathological, is that the patient repeats representational, or behavioural conduct, in spite of the fact that it is harmful to him and/or his environment. This becomes the unique, or at least the preferential reaction, in certain internal or external situations with which the patient is confronted. This restricting characteristic of a behaviour and its propensity to reorganize the personality of the adolescent, depends on two sets of parameters:
– the weight and the nature of factors of vulnerability, but also of factors of self-protection and resilience which are part of the patient's past, family and individual history.

– both the personal and the social context of the adolescent, taking into account events, as well as the way the environment responds to his implicit and explicit expectations.

The conjuncture of all of these parameters is specific to adolescence. For a major part, they remain in a virtual state. The adolescent may put them into play either temporarily, on a long-term basis, or even permanently. We are confronted with a wide scope of possibilities, ranging from situations where the weight of different pathogenic restrictions is such that one or more pathological behaviours are certain to appear, to situations where pathological behaviour will materialize only in accordance with the nature of environmental response.
The symptoms of the patient's restricting disorders, whether they be psychotic, behavioural, addictive, or other, may be more or less completely expressed. The spectrum of interaction of neuro-biological dysfunctioning and purely relational dysfunctioning is very wide and each modality influences the other.
In this perspective, a psychiatric response could be considered as a sort of psychosomatic response to stress, in combination with a breakdown of relational and narcissistic adjustments such as we have briefly described, and whose extent and severity are conditioned by both subjacent neuro-biological vulnerabilities and environmental factors, in varying proportions according to each case.
This theoretical conception corresponds to our clinical experience and induces us to actively combat all the aforementioned types of pathogenic functioning, whether or not they have been diagnosed as psychosis. We intervene with all the possible means at our disposal, from individual, group or family psychotherapy to psychotropic drugs.

Thus we feel that it is necessary to approach psychopathology in a multi-dimensional way. Our therapy is based on the importance of environmental factors in the development of the patient's identity. However, we by no means neglect biological factors. Psychopathologic disorders are potentially inherent in man's specific psychic development, which allows him to attain self-awareness, and confronts him with a fundamental existential paradox: in order to develop, man needs to be resourced by external objects of attachment. Yet this necessity may be experienced as a threat to an equally important need: that of differentiating himself from others and maintaining his identity. This potentiality may give rise to psychic disorders when narcissism, instead of gaining strength from objectal bonds, tries to protect itself from a threat of annihilation by avoiding or even destroying these bonds. Disorders are even more likely to develop if there is a biological vulnerability, inherently non-specific, multi-genetic and multi-factorial, to feelings and handling emotions. The clinical expression of this disorders will vary according to a combination of psychic and environmental factors. This combination of biological, psychic and environmental restrictions is all the more complex in that any symptom, whatever the cause of its appearance, is liable to play a role in organizing the patient's relation to himself and to others.

References

1. Holmes J. Attachment theory: a biological basis for psychotherapy? *Br J Psychiatry* 1993a; 163: 430-8.
2. Shore A. Attachment and the regulation of the right brain. *Attachment & Human Development* 2000; 2: 23-47.
3. Lichtenberg JD. Écouter, comprendre et interpréter. Réflexions sur la complexité. *Psychothérapies* 2004; 24: 55-72.
4. Fonagy P, Target M, Cottrell D, et al. *What works for whom? A critical review of treatments for children and adolescents.* New York: The Guildford Press, 2002.
5. Zeanah C. (ed.). *Handbook of Infant Mental Health.* New York: Guildford Press, 2000.
6. Guedeney N, Guedeney A, Rabouam C, et al. L'utilisation de la classification diagnostique Zero to Three à partir d'une observation. *Prisme* 2000; 33: 80-91.
7. Cramer B. Can therapists learn from psychotherapy research. In: Von Klitzing K, Tyson P, Burgin D, eds. *Psychoanalysis in childhood and adolescence.* Basel: Karger, 2000; 2-22.
8. Holmes J. *The search for a secure base. Attachment theory and psychotherapy.* New York: Routledge, 2001.
9. Fraiberg S. Clinical studies of infant mental health. The first year of life. London: Tavistock Publications, 1980. Trad. Française: Paris: PUF, 1999.
10. Bowlby J. *A secure base.* New York: Basic Books, 1988.
11. Birmaher B, Ryan ND, Williamson DE, et al. Childhood and adolescent depression. A review of the past ten years. Part I. *J Am Acad Child Adolesc Psychiatry* 1996; 35: 1427-39.
12. Fombonne E, Wostear G, Cooper V, et al. The Maudsley long term follow-up of chills and adolescent depression. Suicidality, criminality and social dysfunction in adulthood. *Br J Psychiatry* 2001; 179: 218-23.
13. Lewinsohn PM, Allen NB, Seeley JR, et al. First onset versus recurrence of depression: Differential processes of psychosocial risk. *J Abnorm Psychol* 1999; 108: 483-9.
14. Bardone AM, Moffitt TE, Caspi A, et al. Adult mental health and social outcomes of adolescent girls with depression and conduct disorder. *Dev Psychopathol* 1996; 8: 811-29.
15. Harrington R, Fudge H, Rutter M, et al. Adult outcomes of child and adolescent depression. I. Psychiatric status. *Arch General Psychiatry* 1990; 47: 465-73.
16. Rao U, Dahl RE, Ryan ND, et al. Unipolar depression in adolescents: Clinical outcome in adulthood. *J Am Acad Child Adolesc Psychiatry* 1995; 34: 566-78.
17. Reuter MA, Scaramella L, Wallace LE, et al. First onset of depressive symptoms or anxiety disorder predicted by the longitudinal course of internalizing symptoms and parent-adolescent disagreements. *Arch Gen Psychiatry* 1999; 56: 726-32.
18. Klein DN, Lewinsohn PM, Seeley Jr, et al. A family study of major depressive disorder in a community sample of adolescents. *Arch General Psychiatry* 2001; 58: 13-20.
19. Wickramaratne PJ, Weissman MM. Onset of psychopathology in offspring by developmental phase and parental depression. *J Am Acad Child Adolesc Psychiatry* 1998; 37: 933-42.
20. Birmaher B, Brent DA, Kolko D et al. Clinical outcome after short-term psychotherapy for adolescents with major depressive disorder. *Arch Gen Psychiatry* 2000; 57: 29-36.
21. Brent DA, Holder D, Kolko D et al. A clinical psychotherapy trial for adolescent depression comparing cognitive, family and supportive therapy. *Arch General Psychiatry* 1997; 54: 877-85.
22. Vasquez-Barquero JL, Lastra I, Cuesta Nunez J, et al. Patterns of positive and negative symptoms in first episode schizophrenia. *Br J Psychiatry* 1996; 168: 693-701.
23. Mc Clellan J, Werry J. Practice parameters for the assessment and treatment of children and adolescents with schizophrenia. *J Am Acad Child Adolesc Psychiatry* 1994; 33: 616-35.
24. Yung AR, Mc Gorry PD. The prodromal phase of first-episode psychosis: past and current conceptualizations. *Schizophrenia Bulletin* 1996; 22: 353-70.

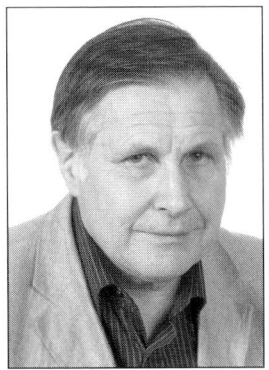

Scientific Advances in Neonatology since the Year 2000*

Hugo LAGERCRANTZ

Karolinska Institute, Astrid Lindgren Hospital for Children, Stockholm, Sweden

Few areas in medicine have been so successful with regard to decreasing mortality as neonatology during the last 50 years. The infant mortality has decreased substantially in nearly all countries of the world. The increase of survival of preterm infants has been staggering in North America and the European Union [1]. The survival of infants with a birthweight less than 1,000 grammes has increased from 10-20% to 80-90% (*figure 1*). Major factors behind this success are improvement of the thermal mileu, better nutrition, oxygen and respiratory support. More specific factors are the introduction of surfactant in clinical practice and stimulation of lung maturation by corticosteroids which were introduced in the 1980s [2,3].

---

* With special reference to some discoveries awarded with the Nobel Prize in Physiology or Medicine.

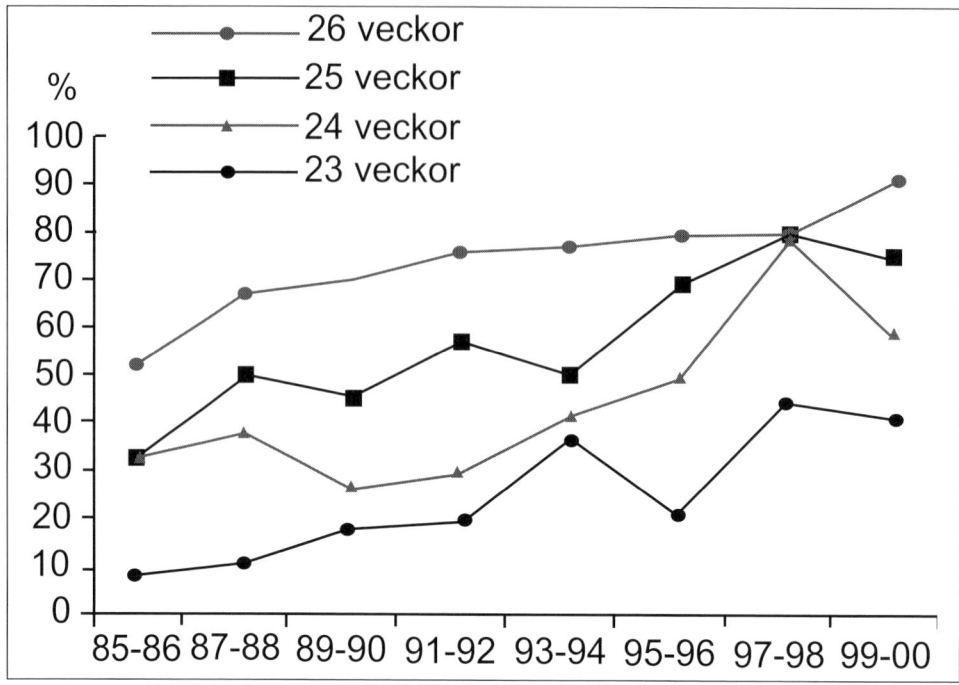

Figure 1. Survival of infants born after 23-26 gestational weeks in Sweden 1985-2000.

Pharmacological agents like dopamine, indomethacin, caffeine and nitric oxide (NO) are also of major importance to improve neonatal outcome. We are now usually able to treat most of the cardiorespiratory diseases of newborn infants. The major problem today is to prevent neurological sequele particularly in severely asphyxiated and extremely preterm infants [4].

An interesting notion is that some advances in progress in neonatology are based on scientific discoveries which have been awarded with the Nobel Prize in physiology or medicine. Major discoveries on the transmission of infections diseases have of course been of great importance to decrease neonatal mortality, like Charles Nicolle's discovery of how typhus is transmitted via lice, which was awarded the Nobel Prize 1928. Four main topics may be of great importance for neonatal medicine at least during the beginning of this century.

Making of the brain

This year we celebrate the centennial of the Nobel prize award to Raymon y Cajal and Camillo Golgi for their discoveries of the construction of the brain. Particularly Cajal investigated the infant brain since *"the full grown forests turns out to be impenetrable and indefinable, why not revert to the study of the young woods in the nursery stage as we may say"* [5].

Hans Spemann received the Prize in 1935 for his discoveries of the organizer of the brain [6].
During recent years we have learned which factors are involved in the induction of the brain. The ectoderm seems to be transformed to neural tissue by a default pathway. However, this transformation is blocked by BMP (brain morphogenic factor). To develop neural tissue BMP has to be antagonized by folin or noggin, which may correspond to the Spemann's organizer [6, 7].
Recent findings on neuronal migration seem to be important. Besides the migration along the radial glia there is a tangential migration of neurons particularly in the human, which results in the great expansion of the human brain and its capacity to deal with symbols and language [8].
These findings are probably of major clinical importance. Disturbances of neuronal migration and wiring may lead to autism and schizophrenia. Viral infections during pregnancy seem to be the major non-genetic cause of autism [9]. Fetuses who are subjected to viral infections [10] or stress seem to have a higher risk of developing schizophrenia particularly if there is heritage for that disease in the family. One possible mechanism to explain these observations may be a distrubance of the expression of major histocompatibility complex (MHC) molecules [11]. These molecules seem to play an important role in the wiring of the neuronal network.

Critical periods and developing care

David Hubel and Torsten Wiesel received the Nobel Prize in physiology or medicine 1981 together with Roger Sperry for their discoveries concerning information processing in the visual system. Of particular interest for neonatal medicine was their explanation of the pathogenesis to amblyopia. They showed that if there is an imbalance of input between the two eyes by closing one eye during the critical period there is a functional shift of the ocular dominance (OD) of cortical neurons in favour of the open eye (*figure 2*). Analyses of the visual cortex showed wider OD columns representing the seeing eye as compared with the blind one. Thus the newborn must use both eyes during a critical period. If not due to cataract or severe squint, the infant will develop cortical blindness corresponding to the affected eye(s).

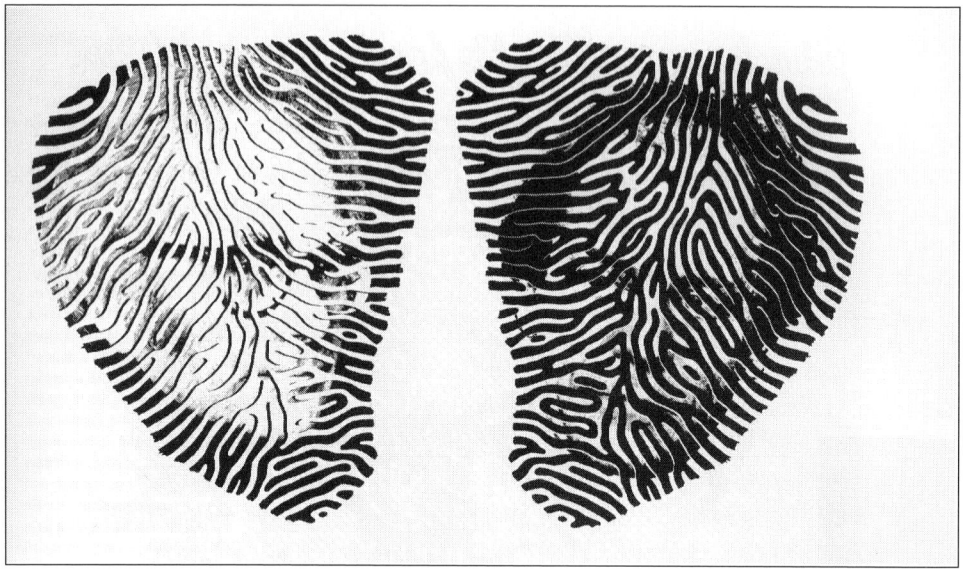

Figure 2. Ocular dominance columns (ODC) in the visual cortex. If one eye is covered in the newborn kitten, the ODC atrofy and appear white (left). The siloultes of the discovereres David Hubel and Torsten Wiesel have been transposed on the patterns (Nicolaus Wade).

The wiring of the neurons and the refinement of the connections are dependent on spontanous nervous activity. This process has been extensively studied in the visual system, where axons from the two eyes form specific layers in the lateral geniculate nucleus. This process involves "*the formation, elimination and reorganization of individual synaptic connections*" [12]. There is a spontanous activity which sweep in wawes over the retina and subsequentially in the visual cortex. If this process is blocked by toxins like tetrodotoxin the ferrets become blind. Thus it is essential that the neurons "*which fire together wire together, those which don't won't!*"

At this stage we can only speculate about the clinical importance of these experimental findings. Very preterm infants are bombared by various inputs from its sensory organs in the neonatal ward. Bright light, voices from the staff and noise from the environment and pain. A preterm infant may be exposed to hundreds of uncomfortable invasions like heel pricks, ultrasound, sucking the throat, intubations etc. We may suspect that extrauterine overstimulation may affect the firing and wiring the neurons. There are studies showing that ex-preterm children have a greater risk of developing attention deficit hyperactivity disorders (ADHD), anxiety, phobias and cognitive deficits [13]. These problems also occur in children who have not suffered from any major CNS catastrophy like intraventricular bleeding.

To prevent neuropsychological sequelae Heidelise Als in Boston has developed a new caring philosophy: Newborn individualized developmental care and assessment program (Nidcap). The idea is to reduce external overstimulation, by covering the incubators with blankets and place the infants in nests simulating the intrauterine milieu (*figure 3*). Furthermore the nurses make frequent observations regarding the autonomic stability of the infant. The number of invasive procedures are reduced and only allowed when the baby is in stable condition. The parents are taught to interpret the signals of the infant. Several studies from North America and Europe have demonstrated improved outcome of infants treated by developmental care as compared with conventional care [14]. In one study it was demonstrated that the myelination seemed to be improved by using diffusion tensor imaging [15].

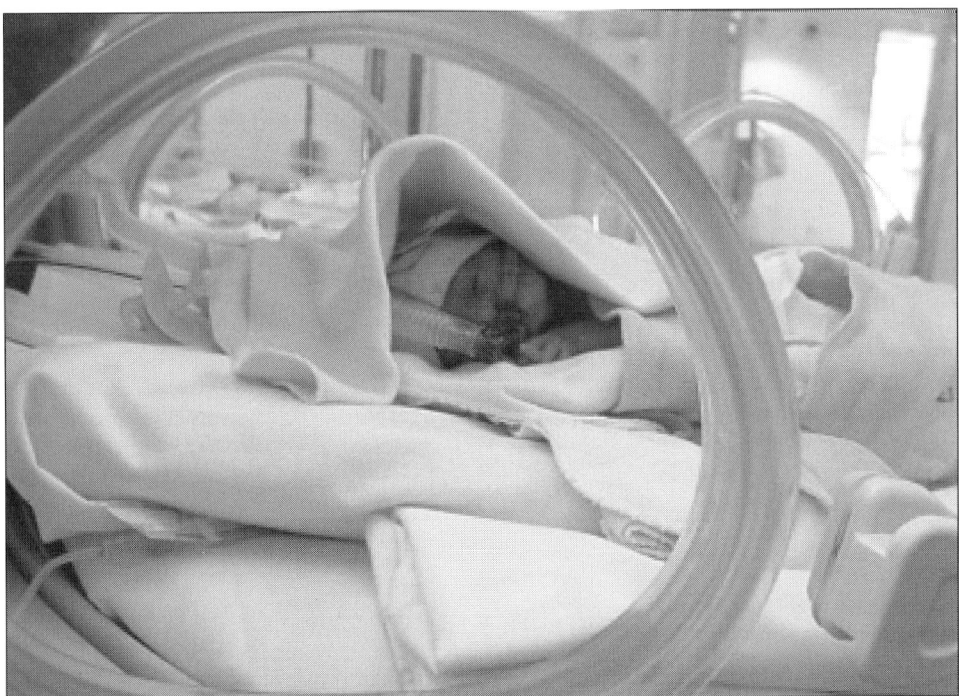

Figure 3. In developmental care the preterm infant is placed in a nest and protected towards environmental stress factors.
Photo by Ann-Sofi Gustafsson.

The long-term outcome of these children was also found to be improved, when these children were tested at three years. The question is whether there is any biological explanation.

Recent studies by Michael Meaney and his group have demonstrated the effect of maternal handling on gene expression [16]. Rat pups which were intensively licked and groomed (LG) by their mothers developed better than those which were not. They demonstrated that LG increased the expression of glucocorticoid receptors in the hippocampus. This resulted in a negative feedback i.e. less release of corticotrophin. When these offsprings were subjected to stress as adults they responded with a lower corticosteroid release. This effect seemed to be mediated by serotonin which may be more released in the high-LG group and susequetly enhance glucocorticoid receptor upregulation (*figure 4*). These important findings may be of relevance for neonatal care. Although there is some controversy regarding the long-term effect of developing care, the mode of neonatal care seem to matter.

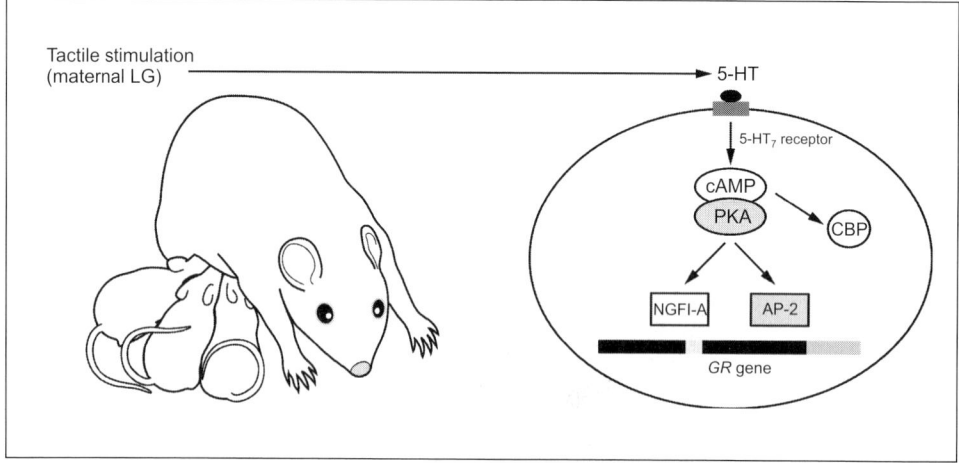

Figure 4. Increased licking and grooming (LG) stimulates serotonin (5-HT) turnover in the hippocampus. This leads to stimulation of the glucocorticoid (GR) receptors. Lack of LG results in less expression of GR receptors and subsequent lower stress tolerance.

Brain imaging

New techniques imaging the brain have revolutionized neonatal medicine. In 1997 the Nobel Prize was jointly awarded to Allan Cormack and Geoffrey Hounsfield for their discovery of the CT scan and in 2003 to Paul Lauterbur and Peter Mansfield for the discovery of magnetic resonance imaging.

By using computerized tomography intraventricular bleedings were surprisingly often detected in preterm infants [17]. Ultrasound was found to be more practical to diagnose cerebral lesions in the nursery. For more sophisticated analyses of brain morphology and pathology MR technique has proved to be very effective [18] (*figure 5*). White matter disease which is now the most common problem in the extremely preterm infants cannot so easily be detected by CT or ultrasound as by MR [19, 20]. By using diffusion tensor imaging (DTI) it is possible to study myelination. MR scanning of preterm infants particularly before they are discharged from the hospital or at follow-up has proved to be very useful to predict longterm outcome. MR scanning of preterm graduates during adolescense has shown that some areas of the brain have smaller volumes than in matched controls [13]. Preterm graduates have also been found to have lower anisotrophy indicating deficient myelination [21].

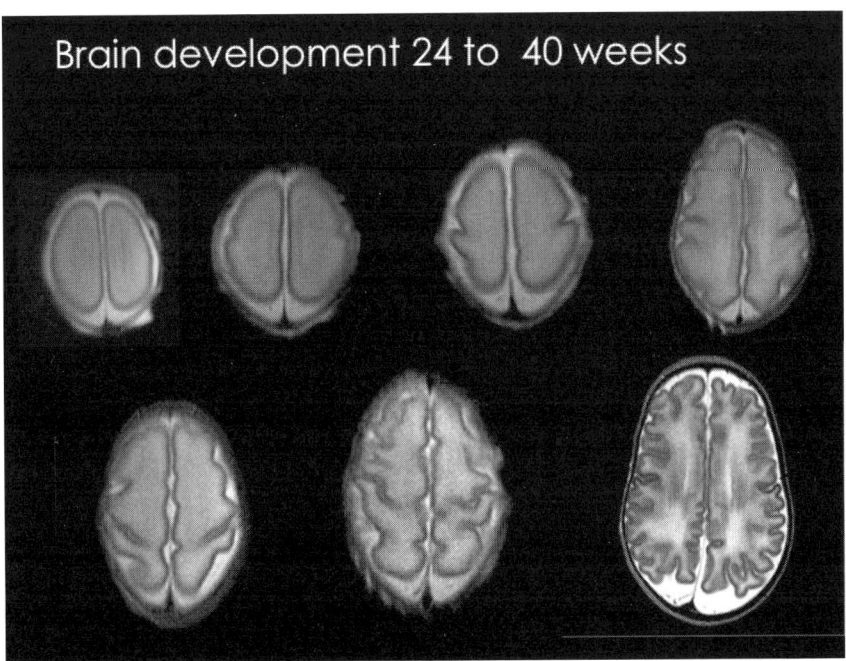

Figure 5. MR images of the neonatal brain of infants born after 24-30 weeks gestational age. From Mary Rutherford, Imperial College, London.

The ultimate goal of brain imaging is to visualize how the baby processes sensory stimulation. How does it perceive viewing its mother's face and hearing her voice? To what extent is the baby conscious about for example pain?

To study this functional MR is necessary. However, it is a little unpractical to perform these studies in babies. A number of studies in adults and older children have given us completely new information on how the brain is processing sensory input like recognizing faces, listening to language and music or perceiving smell, taste and pain. This has been difficult to repeat in babies, since it is necessary that they are kept immobile. However, we have learned a lot about how the baby is processing sensory input by using other techniques like near-infrared-spectroscopy (NIRS). This method is based on the computation of the reflection of near-infra red light by hemoglobin and other chromophobes. In this way it is possible to get a semiquantitative measure of blood flow for example in the olfactory or sensory area [22]. Newborn babies were found to react to smells of milk and vanilla and also bad odours at a cortical level. Recently two groups have independently demonstrated that the sensory cortex is activated by pain in preterm infants, suggesting that they may be aware of pain at a cortical level [23, 24].

Another tool is magnetoencephalography which can filter out movement artifacts. We can certainly expect a number of breakthroughs in our understanding of the infant brain by new imaging techniques.

Chemical transmittors in neonatal medicine

Henry Dale and Otto Loewi were awarded the Nobel Prize 1936 for "their discoveries relating to chemical transmission of nerve impulses". Bernard Katz, Ulf von Euler and Julius Axelrod received the Prize 1970 for "their discoveries concerning the humoral transmitters in the nerve terminal and the mechanism for their storage, release and inactivation".

The main chemical transmittors of significance for neonatal medicine are the catecholamines. Remarkably high amounts of noradrenaline and adrenaline are released in the fetus and the newborn during vaginal delivery. This is probably of importance for neonatal adaptation, since infants delivered by elective caesarean section have lower levels and some problems like wet lungs and hypoglycemia which may be related to their lack of catecholamine surge [25]. Dopamine is extensively used in neonatal medicine to treat hypotension. Disturbances of monoamine turnover during the perinatal period may be related to the development of ADHD and other psychiatric disorders. There are some indications that fetal hypoxia may cause longterm disturbance of monoamine turnover lasting up to adult life [26]. This area of research i.e. developmental programming is now one of the most promising research fields [27].

Sune Bergström, Bengt Samuelsson and John Vane were awarded the Nobel prize 1982 for their discoveries of prostaglandins and related substances. These discoveries have a major impact on reproductive and neonatal medicine. The role of prostaglandins for the patency of the ductus arteriosus is well established as well as treating this condition with antagonists like indomethacin and ibuprofen. Prostaglandins also seem to be of importance suppressing fetal breathing movements. A placental factor inhibiting breathing has recently been identified as a prostaglandin [28]. Interestingly is also that recent studies indicate that indomethacin has a longterm neuroprotective effect particularly in boys [29].

The discovery of nitric oxide (NO) has also a major impact in neonatal medicine. Robert Furchgott discovered a vasodilating substance in the intima of blood vessels (endothelium derived relating factor – EDRF). This factor was then identified by Louis Ignarro as the gas NO. NO seems to be involved in the dilatation of the pulmonary arteries at birth [30]. NO is now the drug of choice to treat persistent pulmonary hypertension of the newborn (PPHN) or persistent fetal circulation. It has markedly reduced the need for extracorporal circulation.

The interesting new development is that NO given to preterm infants seems to prevent the development of bronchopulmonary dysplasia (BPD). NO decreases lung neutrophil accumulation and thus the inflammatory cascade which leads to BPD [31]. Furthermore it also seems to have some neuroprotective role. Follow-up of preterm infants treated with NO has recently shown that these infants develop less neurological sequele than matched controls.

References

1. Horbar JD, Badger GJ, Carpenter JH, *et al*. Trends in mortality and morbidity for very low birth weight infants 1991-1999. *Pediatrics* 2002; 110: 143-51.
2. Ariagno RI, Martin GI, Raju TNK. Neonatology research for the 21st century. *J Perinatology* 2006; 26: S1-S56.
3. Cooke RW. Preterm mortality and morbidity over 25 years. Arch Dis Child Fetal Neonatal 2006; 91: 293-4.
4. Gressens P, Rogida M, Paindaveine B, Sola A. The impact of neonatal intensive care practices on the developing brain. *J Pediatrics* 2002; 140: 646-53.
5. Lagercrantz H. Nobel Prizes in paediatrics: Santiago Ramon y Cajal (1852-1934) and the founding of neuroembryology. *Acta Paediatr.* 2006; 95: 130-1.
6. Lagercrantz H. Hans Spemann: discoverer of the neuronal organizer. *Acta Paediatr* 2006; 95: 386-7.
7. Jessell TM, Sanes JR. The decade of the developing brain. *Curr Opin Neurobiology* 2000; 10: 599-611.
8. Letinic K, Zoncu R, Rakic P.Origin of GABAergic neurons in the human neocortex. *Nature* 2002; 417: 645-9.
9. Ciaranello AL, Ciaranello RD.The neurobiology of infantile autism. *Annu Rev Neurosci* 1995; 18: 101-28.
10. Stefan MD, Murray RM. Schizophrenia: developmental disturbance of brain and mind? *Acta Paediatr* 1997; 422: S112-S116.

11. Boulanger LM, Shatz CJ. Immune signalling in neural development, synaptic plasticity and disease. *Nat Rev Neurosci* 2004; 5: 521-31.
12. Katz Lc, Shatz CJ. Synaptic activity and the construction of cortical circuits. *Science* 1996; 274: 1133-8.
13. Ment LR, Vohr B, Allan W, et al. Change in cognitive function over time in very low-birthweight infants. *JAMA* 2003; 289: 705-11.
14. Sizun J, Browne JV. *Research on early developmental care for preterm neonates*. Paris: John Libey Eurotext, 2005.
15. Als H, Duffy FH, McAnulty GB, et al. Early experience alters brain function and structure. *Pediatrics* 2004; 113: 846-57.
16. Meaney MJ, Szyf M. Maternal care as a model for experience-dependent chromatin plasticity? *Trends Neurosci* 2005; 28: 456-63.
17. Fitzhardinge PM, Flodmark O, Fitz CR, Ashby S. The prognostic value of computed tomography of the brain in asphyxiated premature infants. *J Pediatr* 1982;100: 476-81.
18. Ment LR, Bada HS, Barnes P, et al. Practice parameter: neuroimaging of the neonate: report of the Quality Standards Subcommittee of the American Academy of Neurology and the Practice Committee of the Child Neurology Society. *Neurology* 2002; 58: 1726-38.
19. Huppi PS. Immature white matter lesions in the premature infant. *J Pediatr* 2004; 145: 575-8.
20. Inder TE, Warfield SK, Wang H, et al. Abnormal cerebral structure is present at term in premature infants. *Pediatrics* 2005; 115: 286-94.
21. Nagy Z, Westerberg H, Skare S, et al. Preterm children have disturbances of white matter at 11 years of age as shown by diffusion tensor imaging. *Pediatr Res* 2003; 54: 672-9.
22. Bartocci M, Winberg J, Papendieck G, et al. Cerebral hemodynamic response to unpleasant odors in the preterm newborn measured by near-infrared spectroscopy. *Pediatric Research* 2001; 50: 324-30.
23. Fitzgerald M. The development of nociceptive circuits. *Nature Rev Neurosci* 2006; 6: 507-19.
24. Bartocci M, Bergqvist LL, Lagercrantz H, Anand KJ. Pain activates cortical areas in the preterm newborn brain. *Pain*. 2006; 122: 109-17.
25. Lagercrantz H, Slotkin T. The stress of being born. *Sci Am* 1986; 254: 100-10.
26. Peyronnet J, Roux JC, Geloën A, et al. Prenatal hypoxia impairs the postnatal development of neural and functional chemoafferent pathway in rat. *J Physiol* 2000; 524: 525-37.
27. Barker DJ. Fetal origins of cardiovascular disease. *Ann Med* 1999; 31: 3-6.
28. Alvaro RE, Hasan SU, Chemtob S, et al. Prostaglandins are responsible for the inhibition of breathing observed with a placental extract in fetal sheep. *Respir Physiol Neurobiol* 2004.
29. Ment LR, Peterson BS, Meltzer JA, et al. A functional magnetic resonance imaging study of the long-term influences of early indomethacin exposure on language processing in the brains of prematurely born children. *Pediatrics* 2006: 118: 961-7.
30. Rairigh RL, Parker TA, Ivy DD, et al. Role of inducible nitric oxide synthase in the pulmonary vascular response to birth-related stimuli in the ovine fetus. *Circ Res* 2001; 88: 721-6.
31. Kinsella JP: Inhaled nitric oxide therapy in premature newborn. *Curr Opin Pediatr* 2006; 18: 107-11.

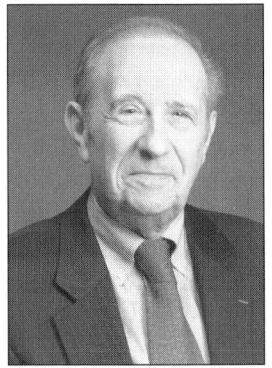

Present and Future in Vaccinology*

Stanley PLOTKIN

*University of Pennsylvania, Philadelphia, PA, USA
and Sanofi Pasteur, Lyon, France*

Immunization is now two hundred years old.

The history of vaccines began with the work of Jenner, who observed that vaccinia protected against smallpox. But it was Pasteur's work in the 1880s that enabled definition of the principles underlying immunization and inaugurated vaccinology with the development of the first rabies vaccine for humans. In the first half of the 20th century, new methods of attenuating virulence through passaging in animals, eggs or *in vitro* led to the development of BCG vaccine and yellow fever vaccine. After the Second World War, with the discovery of virus growth in cell culture, numerous other attenuated live vaccines were developed: measles, poliomyelitis and mumps; then later, varicella, rubella and influenza vaccines. Concomitantly, Inactivated vaccines were developed for typhoid, cholera, and plague late in the

---

* Article written by Dr Hélène Collignon for *Médecine et Enfance* and translated by Professor Stanley Plotkin.

immunized subjects presented with clinical disease versus 21% of the subjects in the control group. Recent results with the vaccine, which has undergone large-scale clinical development, show that it induces 98% protection against severe gastroenteritis and 74% protection against all forms of the disease.

Third lesson: natural immunity is generally superior to vaccine-induced immunity

This has clearly been shown by a study on cytomegalovirus conducted a few years ago. Cytomegalovirus is the main infectious cause of mental retardation and congenital deafness and work on developing a vaccine is ongoing. Three doses of wild virus were tested as a challenge: 10, 100 and 1,000 PFU. For seronegative subjects, the 10 PFU dose level was sufficient to induce infection, but in seropositive subjects, i.e. those who had already experienced an infection, only the 1,000 PFU dose induced infection. Vaccinated subjects were protected against the 100 PFU dose, but not against the 1,000 PFU dose. These results clearly show the power of natural immunity and its superiority to vaccinal immunity.

Fourth lesson: it is relatively difficult to immunize infants and the elderly

Maternal antibodies are known to interfere with immunization of infants. That is why, for instance, infants are not vaccinated against measles until they are 12 months old. Moreover, even when the infant no longer has maternal antibodies, the immune system remains immature. A study which included infants of various ages who no longer had maternal antibodies showed that at 12 months of age, the response to measles immunization was excellent, while at 9 months of age the response was weak and weaker still at 6 months (*figure 1*).

The development of conjugated bacterial polysaccharide vaccines has now enabled infants to be immunized against *Haemophilus influenzae* type b, pneumococcus and meningococcus as of two months of age. The conjugated meningococcus vaccine, for example, has multiple advantages: it induces a higher antibody titer; it elicits immune memory in young children; and it reduces microorganism carriage in the throat. However, we also know that, without a booster, the efficacy of the vaccine in infants declines sharply.

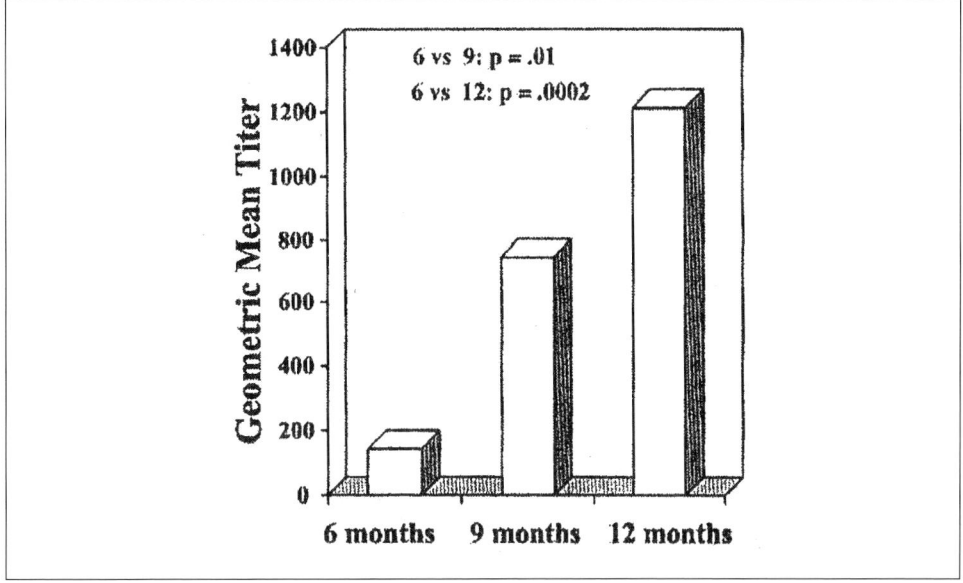

Figure 1. Measles antibody response in infants without maternal antibodies.
Gans *et al.* Vacine 21, 2003: 3398-3405.

There are five main groups of meningococcus pathogenic to man: A, B, C, W135 and Y. A quadrivalent (A, C, W135 and Y) conjugated vaccine is available in the United States and is widely administered to adolescents and students. No conjugated vaccine for group B has been developed because the capsule proteins of meningococcus group B have a degree of homology with a human brain glycoprotein. Other strategies have therefore been adopted in order to develop a group B vaccine. Initially, bacterial external membrane proteins were used. In a study conducted in Brazil, the efficacy of one such vaccine was, once again, shown to be very weak in infants less than two years of age, partial in older children and more marked in schoolchildren. The experiments were nonetheless a success in that the vaccines were shown to halt meningococcal infection epidemics. The same type of vaccine was recently used in New Zealand, a country which has experienced a large epidemic of meningococcus group B infections. Immunization very rapidly induced a marked decrease in the incidence of infection. In the future, another strategy, reverse vaccinology, should enable development of an even more effective meningococcus B vaccine. The method is based on sequencing the bacterial genome (about 600 genes for group B) to identify genes coding for surface proteins with the ability to induce production of neutralizing antibodies. The immunogenicity and protection induced by the proteins are then evaluated in mice. A vaccine could then be based on several of the proteins, providing that they are conserved, i.e. present on all the bacterial strains. This approach has now made considerable progress and we can expect a new meningococcus group B vaccine to become available.

At the other age extreme, in the elderly, immunity is also less powerful. The influenza vaccine, for example, which is about 80% effective against severe forms of the infection in young adults, is only 48% effective with respect to preventing hospitalization and 50% effective in preventing mortality in the elderly. We are currently unable to slow the aging of the immune system, which is related to exhaustion of naïve B- and T-cells.

Fifth lesson: the functional characteristics of antibodies are as important as their quantity

The example of the pneumococcal polysaccharide vaccine administered to the elderly provides a good illustration. After vaccination, antibody response may be evaluated in two ways: by an ELISA to detect antibodies bound to antigens and by a functional test to determine phagocytic capability in which a serum sample from the immunized subject is exposed to the bacterium responsible for the infection. Subjects aged over 60 years produce antibodies that are detectable by ELISA, but, compared to young subjects, relatively few functional antibodies. This explains why a vaccine that is highly effective in young subjects may only have moderate efficacy in the elderly.

Sixth lesson: Herd immunity increases with the efficacy of vaccines in the field

In other words, the efficacy of immunization derives not only from the protection conferred on an individual by the vaccine, but also the collective immunity related to blocking propagation of the pathogen. This herd immunity also protects unvaccinated subjects. In the United States, administration of pneumococcal vaccine to all children gave rise to a spectacular reduction in invasive infections. A further consequence was a very marked reduction (55%) in infections due to the vaccinal serotypes in adults living in contact with immunized children.

The future

New strategies for vaccine development are being defined and will be increasingly implemented in the future: reassortment of genomic RNA segments, reverse genetics, recombination, replication, defective viruses and DNA plasmids, to mention but a few (*Table 2*). But with regard to the future the most important point is that molecular biology has opened the way for development of vaccines for almost all diseases, provided, of course, that the pathogenesis of the disease has been elucidated.

Table 2. Newer strategies for vaccine development

Reassortment of RNA genome segments
Reverse genetics and ts mutations
Replicating agents recombined with genes from pathogens
Replication - Defective particles
Replication - Defective viruses or bacteria
DNA plasmids
Reverse vaccinology
Recombinant proteins genetically inactivated
Fusion proteins
Gene delivery by invasive bacteria
Combination vaccines

The reassortment method has been used to develop a new live influenza virus for administration by the nasal route. In addition to the fact that the nasal route simplifies vaccine administration, the vaccine confers a broader immunity. The vaccine not only induces strong immunity when the vaccinal viral strain and that circulating are the same, but also when they are different. This is not usually observed with an inactivated vaccine. A study conducted in two cities in Texas showed that immunization of children in their schools not only reduced the immunized childrens' absences from school and visits to their physicians, it also reduced adult sick leave and consultations. The protection conferred on adults through the immunization of children is related to a reduction in the number of influenza virus carriers induced by the immunization.

Recombination, another new strategy for vaccine development, has been used to develop an as yet investigational parainfluenza virus vaccine. The latter virus is associated with respiratory tract infections that are potentially serious in young children. The method enabled development of a recombinant vaccine for the three types of parainfluenza virus. Recombination has also been used to develop a respiratory syncytial virus vaccine by placing the gene for the RSV F protein in the attenuated parainfluenza strain. The vaccine has already been shown to be effective in animals and is currently under clinical development.

An important recent strategy is the use of non-pathogenic vectors to carry genes from pathogens. Although there is not yet a licensed human vaccine based on vectors, adenoviruses and poxviruses vectors are prominent in experimental vaccinology for such diseases as AIDS. They are particularly useful in the induction of cellular immune responses.

Lastly, a major breakthrough in the field of immunization was recently achieved: development of a human papillomavirus (HPV) vaccine, also using the methods of molecular biology. Papillomavirus infection is sexually transmitted and affects 50% of women at some time in their lives. While infection is usually transient, if it persists it may induce cervical dysplasia and cervical cancer. Two HPV vaccines have been shown to procure virtually 100% protection against the two major serotypes causing cancer. They should enable prevention of 70% of cervical cancers.

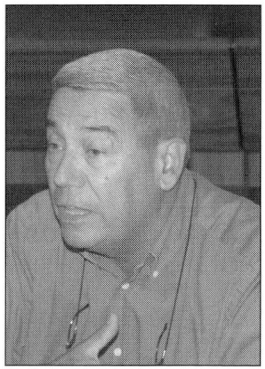

Clinical Approach to Inborn Metabolic Diseases: an Update

Jean-Marie SAUDUBRAY

Consultant in hereditary metabolic diseases,
Hôpital Necker, Paris, France

In view of the major improvements in treatment it has become increasingly important that in order for first-line physicians not to miss a treatable disorder, they are able to initiate a simple method of clinical screening, particularly in the emergency room. We present a simplified classification of treatable inborn errors of metabolism (IEM) in 3 groups. Group 1 includes inborn errors (IE) of intermediary metabolism which give rise to an acute or chronic intoxication. It encompasses aminoacidopathies, organic acidurias (OA), urea cycle disorders (UCD), sugar intolerances, metal disorders and porphyrias. Among aminoacidopathies, inborn errors of amino acid synthesis (glutamine synthetase deficiency and defective serine synthesis) are presented. Most of these disorders are treatable. Among them, several new mechanisms of B6-responsive disorders have been recently elucidated and are shown. Group 2 includes IE of intermediary metabolism which affect the cytoplasmic and mitochondrial energetic processes. Cytoplasmic defects encompass those affecting glycolysis, glycogenosis, gluconeogenesis and hyperinsulinisms. Two new groups have been recently described and are presented: cerebral creatine and pentose phosphate pathways defects. Mitochondrial defects include respiratory chain disorders, Krebs cycle and pyruvate oxidation defects, and disorders of fatty acid oxidation and ketone bodies. The first inborn error of coenzyme Q synthesis has been recently described. Group 3 involves cellular organelles and include lysosomal, peroxisomal, glycosylation, and cholesterol synthesis defects. Among these, some lysosomal disorders can be efficiently treated by enzyme replacement or substrate reduction therapies. Congenital disorders of glycosylation (CDG) and cholesterol synthesis defects are presented.

The recent application of tandem mass spectrometry (tandem MS) to newborn screening and prenatal diagnosis has enabled pre-symptomatic diagnosis for some IEM. However, for most the clinical diagnosis of IEM still relies mandatory before sophisticated biochemical investigations.

Introduction

Some 50 years after the first nutritional treatment of phenylketonuria (PKU) and 30 years after the publication of the first book entirely devoted to the treatment of inborn errors of metabolism [1], the 42nd annual symposium of the Society for the study of inborn errors of metabolism, held in Paris on September 2005, was dedicated to treatment of inborn errors of metabolism as the main theme [2]. During the last half century, many new disorders have been discovered and many therapeutic procedures have been tried. Some of these are well established and life-saving; others are still experimental. The long-term outcome of our oldest patients who have already reached adulthood must question our methods for diagnosis, management and treatment. The new field of adult metabolic medicine also raises many new therapeutic problems including the management of pregnancy in affected mothers. Finally our technical ability to undertake systematic neonatal screening for many metabolic disorders raises a number of ethical issues. This chapter presents a simplified classification of treatable inborn errors of metabolism and focuses on new treatable disorders. Given the very important therapeutic progresses, it becomes more and more important to initiate a simple method of clinical screening by the first line physicians with the goal "do not miss a treatable disorder", in particular at the emergency room. The clinical diagnosis of IEM relies upon a small number of important principles:

– In the appropriate clinical context, consider an IEM in parallel with other more common conditions.

– Be aware of symptoms that persist and remain unexplained after the initial treatment and the usual investigations have been performed for more common disorders may be due to IEM.

- Do not confuse a symptom or a syndrome (such as Reye syndrome, Leigh syndrome, sudden infant death, etc.) with an aetiology – the underlying cause may be an IEM yet to be defined.
- Remember that an IEM can present at any age, from fetal life to old age.
- Be aware that although most genetic metabolic errors are hereditary and transmitted as recessive disorders, the majority of individual cases appear sporadic.
- Initially consider IEMs which are amenable to treatment.
- First provide care for the patient (emergency treatment) and then the family (genetic advice).
- Ask help from specialized centres.

Classification of inborn errors

Pathophysiology

From a therapeutic perspective, metabolic disorders can be divided into the following 3 useful groups.

Group 1: Disorders which give rise to intoxication

This group includes inborn errors of intermediary metabolism that lead to an acute or progressive intoxication from the accumulation of toxic compounds proximal to the metabolic block. In this group are the inborn errors of amino acid catabolism (phenylketonuria, maple syrup urine disease, homocystinuria, tyrosinemia, etc.), most organic acidurias (methylmalonic, propionic, isovaleric, etc.), congenital urea cycle defects, sugar intolerances (galactosemia, hereditary fructose intolerance), metal intoxication (Wilson, Menkes, hemochromatosis), and porphyrias. All the conditions in this group share clinical similarities: they do not interfere with the embryo-fetal development and they present with a symptom-free interval and clinical signs of "intoxication", which may be acute (vomiting, coma, liver failure, thromboembolic complications, etc.) or chronic (failure to thrive, developmental delay, ectopia lentis, cardiomyopathy, etc.). Circumstances that can provoke acute metabolic attacks include catabolism, fever, intercurrent illness and food intake. Clinical expression is often both late in onset and intermittent. Most of these disorders are treatable and require the emergency removal of the toxin by special diets, extra-corporeal procedures, or "cleansing" drugs (carnitine, sodium benzoate, penicillamine, vitamins, etc.). Nutritional therapy is the backbone of the treatment in this group. It includes approaches to deplete the toxic substrate that accumulates or replace the crucial metabolic product that is deficient. Breast milk can still play an important role in these special diets. The long-term consequences of artificial diets on the offspring will have to be evaluated particularly as regards possible mechanisms of metabolic imprinting [3]. Strategies to decrease the concentration of toxic substrates or its precursors also involve the administration of a variety of cleansing drugs that would bind the accumulated metabolites and allow their excretion. Pharmacological doses of vitamins have also shown remarkable efficiency in vitamin-responsive disorders.

B6-responsive disorders: pyridoxal-5'-phosphate (pyridoxal-P), the coenzyme form of vitamin B6, is the cofactor for numerous enzymes involved in neurotransmitter metabolism. Pyridoxal-P can be formed from pyridoxine or pyridoxamine by the action of two enzymes, a kinase: pyridoxal kinase (PK) and an oxidase: pyridox(am)ine-5'-phosphate oxidase (PNPO). Formation of pyridoxal-P from dietary pyridoxal or dietary pyridoxal-P (which is hydrolyzed prior to absorption by intestinal phosphatase or tissue non specific alkaline phosphatase) requires only PK. Two inborn disorders involving pyridoxine and pyridoxal phosphate have been recently elucidated [4]. In pyridoxine responsive epilepsy (first reported in 1954) [5], the molecular defect has been recently shown to be due to antiquitin mutations [6]. This protein is functioning as a dehydrogenase of D-1-piperideine-6 dicarboxylic acid (P6C) and 2-aminoadipic acid 6-semialdehyde (α-AASA) on the lysine catabolic pathway. Children with pyridoxine dependent epilepsy (PDE) have increased concentrations of α-AASA and pipecolic acid in CSF, plasma and urine that persist even in B6 treated patients. Mutations in the *ALDH7A1* gene have been identified. Thus PDE is explained by the fact that a defect in the lysine catabolism pathway in the brain leads to accelerated loss of pyridoxal phosphate, the active form of vitamin B6 that reacts with P6C by a Knoevenagel condensation reaction and thus inactivates it. The diagnosis of PDE is now based not only on the B6-responsive test but also on the presence of abnormal metabolites in urine, plasma and CSF even in patients on treatment.

Another group of neonates presents seizures with burst-suppression associated with parkinsonism, hypothermia and hypotonia only responsive to pyridoxal phosphate and not to pyridoxine. In this disorder, CSF concentrations of the dopamine metabolite, HVA, and the serotonine metabolite, 5HIAA, are low. The CSF concentration of the L-dopa metabolite, 3-O-methyl-dopa (also known as 3-methoxytyrosine), are very high. The urinary excretion of another L-dopa metabolite, vanillactic acid, is increased. These changes indicate a reduced activity of the pyridoxal-P dependent enzyme aromatic L-amino acid decarboxylase. Slightly raised CSF concentrations of glycine and threonine are also present and are explained by a reduced activity of the pyridoxal-P dependent glycine cleavage enzyme and threonine dehydratase respectively. This complex metabolic pattern is due to the defective transformation of pyridoxine into its active pyridoxal phosphate cofactor by inherited defect of pyridox(am)ine-P oxidase (PNPO) [7]. In clinical practice, a tentative diagnosis of PNPO deficiency can be made if a neonate has seizures that dramatically respond to pyridoxal-P having failed to respond to pyridoxine. It must be stressed that therapeutic trials must be undertaken with great care as 50 mg of pyridoxal phosphate can lead to cessation of seizures within an hour but sometimes be associated with profound hypotonia and unresponsiveness and also some hypotension [8].

Homocystinuria (cystathionine-b-synthase deficiency) (CBS) is an already well known B6-responsive disorder. Approximately 50% of CBS deficient patients show a marked or a partial response to pyridoxine *in vivo*. An interesting observation that suggests the possibility of a chaperon action of PLP came from the measurement of CBS activity in liver biopsies from patients taken before and after *in vivo* B6 supplementation. The B6 administration lead to 1.3 to 4.5 fold increase in the hepatic CBS activity [9].

Although the pathophysiology is somewhat different from inborn errors of amino acid catabolism, the inborn errors of neurotransmitter synthesis and catabolism (monoamines, GABA and glycine) and the inborn errors of amino acid synthesis (serine, glutamine, and proline/ornithine) can also be included in the group of "intoxication disorders" since they share many characteristics: they are inborn errors of intermediary metabolism, their diagnosis relies on plasma, urine, and CSF investigations (amino acid, organic acid analyses, etc.), and some are amenable to treatment even when the disorder starts *in utero*, like 3-phosphoglycerate dehydrogenase deficiency [10].

3-phosphoglycerate dehydrogenase deficiency has been described in 9 patients belonging to 4 families [11, 12]. They presented at birth with microcephaly and developed pronounced psychomotor retardation, severe spastic tetraplegia, nystagmus and intractable seizures (including hypsarrhythmia). Magnetic resonance imaging of the brain revealed cortical and subcortical hypotrophy and evidence of disturbed myelination. Diagnosis relies on the finding of decreased concentrations of serine and, to a lesser extent, of glycine in CSF and in fasting plasma, due to 3-phosphoglycerate dehydrogenase deficiency, the first step of serine biosynthesis. Serine thus becomes an essential amino acid in these patients. The deficiency of brain serine seems to be the main determinant of the disease as serine plays a major role in the synthesis of important brain and myelin constituents such as proteins, glycine, cysteine, serine phospholipids, sphingomyelins and cerebrosides. The diagnosis is confirmed by finding a deficient activity of 3-phosphoglycerate dehydrogenase in fibroblasts and molecular analysis. Oral L-serine treatment (up to 600 mg/kg/day) in 6 divided doses corrects the biochemical abnormalities, abolishes the convulsions in most patients, even in those in whom many antiepileptic treatment regimens had failed previously. During treatment with L-serine a marked increase in the white matter volume was observed with a progression of myelination. Interestingly in a girl diagnosed prenatally because of decelerating head growth, L-serine given to the mother normalized fetal head growth with subsequent normal psychomotor development on treatment. This is the first example of treatable congenital microcephaly [12].

Glutamine synthetase deficiency is another new inborn error of amino acid synthesis [13, 14]. Glutamine synthetase (GS) is ubiquitously expressed in human tissues, being involved in ammonia detoxification and interorgan nitrogen flux. Inherited systemic deficiency of glutamine secondary to a defect of glutamine synthetase was recently described in two newborns with an early fatal course of disease. Glutamine was virtually absent in their serum, urine and cerebrospinal fluid. One patient was born at 35 weeks after a pregnancy marked by a polyhydramnios associated with micromelia, enlarged cerebral ventricules, a paraventricular cyst, cerebral and cerebellar atrophy with an almost complete agyria. He had a very poor neurological condition, marked axial hypotonia, convulsions, and he died at 2 days of life with cardiac failure. The second patient presented on the first day of life with convulsions and respiratory failure, and developed generalized erythematous rash with blistering of the entire skin. Brain MRI showed delayed gyration, marked white matter change and subependymal cysts. The patient died at 4 weeks from multiple organ failure. Both patients presented absence of glutamine (2 µmol/l in serum, ND in urine, 11 µmol/l in CSF; normal range = 350-880). Ammonia was only slightly elevated in one patient (140 µmol/l). Glutamine synthetase measured in immortalized lymphocytes displayed an almost 0 residual activity. Mutation analysis showed homozygocity for mutations in exon 6 of the GS gene. These interesting observations emphasize for the first time the crucial neuroprotective role of glutamine in the central nervous system and open a new area in the list of inherited disorders giving rise to severe brain malformations. This disorder is unfortunately not treatable at the present time.

Group 2: Disorders involving energy metabolism

These consist of inborn errors of intermediary metabolism with symptoms due at least partly to a deficiency in energy production or utilization within liver, myocardium, muscle, brain or other tissues. This group can be divided into mitochondrial and cytoplasmic energy defects. Mitochondrial defects are the most severe. They encompass the congenital lactic acidemias (defects of pyruvate transporter, pyruvate carboxylase, pyruvate dehydrogenase, and the Krebs cycle), and mitochondrial respiratory chain disorders which are in general not amenable to treatment with the exception of coenzyme Q10 synthesis defect [15], PDH and PC deficiency [16], and the fatty acid oxidation and ketone body defects which are partly treatable.

Cytoplasmic energy defects are generally less severe. In addition to well known disorders of glycolysis, glycogen metabolism and gluconeogenesis, they include the cytoplasmic and mitochondrial metabolic causes of hyperinsulinism, the more recently described disorders of creatine metabolism, of glucose transporters, and the new inborn errors of the pentose phosphate pathway. Some of the mitochondrial disorders and pentose phosphate pathway defects can interfere with the embryo-fetal development and give rise to dysmorphism, dysplasia and malformations [17, 18].

Creatine deficiency syndromes (CDS) are a novel group of inborn errors of creatine synthesis and transport including autosomal recessive argine: glycine amidino transferase (AGAT) and guanidine acetate methyltransferase (GAMT) deficiencies, and the X-linked creatine transporter (SCL6A8) deficiency. In all these disorders the common clinical hallmark is mental retardation, expressive speech delay and epilepsy. The common biochemical hallmark is cerebral creatine deficiency as detected by proton magnetic resonance spectroscopy (H-MRS). Increased levels of guanidine acetic acid (GAA) in body fluids are pathognomonic for GAMT deficiency whereas these levels are reduced in AGAT deficiency. An increased urinary creatine to creatinine ratio is associated with SLC6A8 deficiency. Oral supplementation of creatine leads to partial restauration of the cerebral creatine pool and improvement of clinical symptoms in GAMT and AGAT deficiencies. Reduction of GAA by additional dietary restriction of arginine appears to be of additional benefit for GAMT deficient patients. For SLC6A8 deficient patients, no effective treatment is currently available. CDS may account for a considerable fraction of children and adults with mental retardation (mostly X-linked) of unknown cause and therefore screening for these disorders (by urinary plasma metabolites, brain H-MRS and DNA approach) should be included in the investigation of these populations.

Disorders of glucose transport (GLUT1 and GLUT2 deficiencies): Beside the already well known glucose/galactose malabsorption and renal glycosuria, two other glucose transport disorders have been more recently described, the glucose transporter deficiency syndrome (GLUT1 deficiency) and the Fanconi Bickel syndrome (GLUT2 deficiency) (figure 1).

GLUT1 deficiency syndrome [19, 20] typically presents as an early onset epileptic encephalopathy in the first year of life as cerebral glucose demand increases. Seizures are of various types and frequency, often refractory to anticonvulsants, and sometimes aggravated by fasting. In infants, peculiar eye movements, staring spells, drop attacks and cyanotic spells are frequent. A global developmental delay and a complex motor disorder become apparent in early childhood. Abnormal behaviour and agitation improved by glucose ingestion is frequently observed but is badly interpreted as no obvious hypoglycaemia is found. The diagnosis is based on the finding of hypoglycorrachia (< 45 mg/dl) in the absence of systemic hypoglycaemia and of a central nervous system infection. CSF to blood glucose ratio is superior to the absolute con-

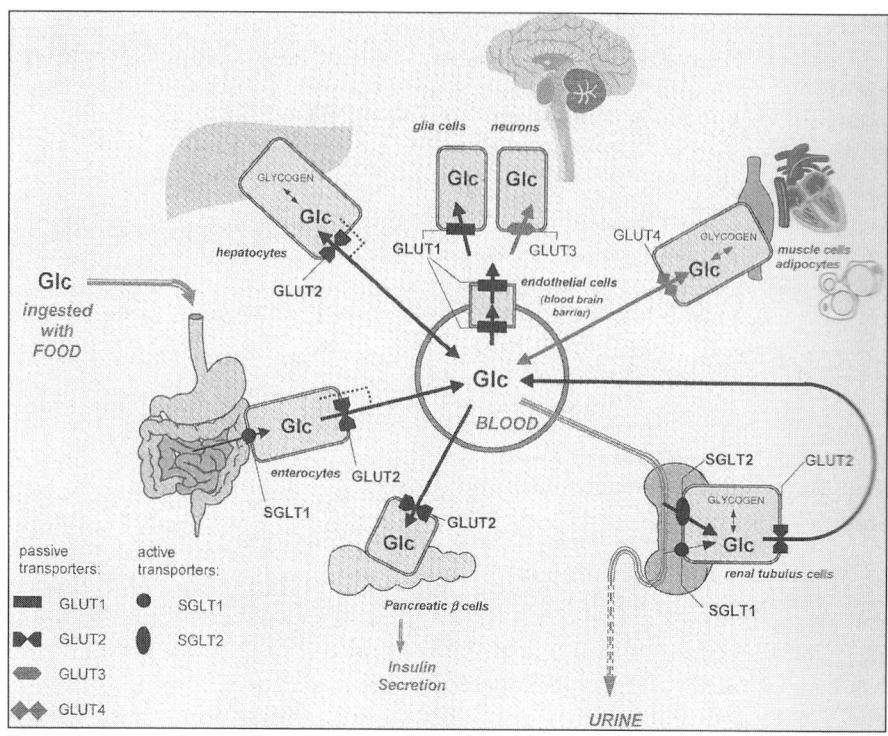

Figure 1. Glucose transporters.

centration in a sample obtained in a non ictal metabolic steady state following a 4-6 hour fast with blood glucose determined before the lumbar puncture to avoid stress-related hyperglycemia. GLUT1 deficiency syndrome should then be confirmed by molecular genetic methods or by glucose uptake studies into erythrocytes (reduced to about half of the control values). GLUT1 is a membrane spanning glycosylated protein that exclusively facilitates glucose transport across the blood brain barrier. GLUT1 also supplies glucose to neurones and glial cells and is the principal fuel for cerebral energy metabolism. Treatment relies on a ketogenic diet throughout childhood and adolescence by which time the cerebral glucose demand decreases to adult levels. Anti convulsant drugs are in general not necessary and even contraindicated (phenobarbital, diazepam which can interfere with GLUT1 function).

Fanconi Bickel syndrome is another well known entity which has been recently shown to be due to GLUT2 deficiency [21, 22].

Inborn errors of the pentose phosphate pathway: The pentose phosphate pathway is present in most cell types. Its function is twofold: the provision of ribose-5-phosphate for ribonucleic acid synthesis and the reduction of NADP into NADPH, a cofactor involved in many biosynthetic processes. Glucose-6-phosphate dehydrogenase is the first irreversible step of the pathway which has been known for a long time, mostly presenting with drug and fava-bean induced haemolytic anaemia. Two other disorders of this pathway have been recently described, the deficiency of ribose-5-phosphate isomerase and the deficiency of transaldolase.

The only patient with ribose-5-phosphate isomerase deficiency presented with developmental and speech delay and epilepsy [23]. From the age of 7 years he regressed with deterioration of vision, speech and walking. At 20 years, he presented spasticity, optic atrophy, nystagmus, cerebellar ataxia, dysarthria and peripheral neuropathy. Brain MRI showed extensive abnormalities of the cerebral white matter with prominent involvement of the U fibres and an abnormal peak of arabitol and ribitol at the brain MRS. Ribose-5-phosphate isomerase deficiency involves the reversible part of the pentose phosphate pathway leading to a decreased capacity to interconvert ribulose-5-phosphate and ribose-5-phosphate resulting in the accumulation of ribose and ribitol (from ribose-5-phosphate) and xylulose and arabitol (from ribulose-5-phosphate). These diagnostic compounds are highly elevated in urines and CSF (tandem mass spectroscopy). The diagnosis can be confirmed by an enzyme assay in fibroblasts and molecular analysis. There is no treatment available.

Transaldolase deficiency is a newly recognised metabolic disease which has been reported so far in 6 patients presenting with liver failure and cirrhosis [18, 24]. All patients presented at birth or in the antenatal period with dysmorphic features, cutis laxa and hypertrichosis, hepatosplenomegaly, hepatic failure, haemolytic anaemia, thrombopenia and genito-urinary malformations. One pregnancy was medically terminated at 28 weeks of gestation because of hydrops fetalis with oligoamnios. The clinical course of the living patients was variable, from early infantile death to an almost complete disappearance of acute liver, cutaneous and haematological findings but leaving a liver fibrosis and a mild renal failure. Diagnosis is based on polyols assessment in urine (tandem MS) that shows elevation of erythritol, arabitol and ribitol. Transaldolase (TALDO) activity is undetectable in the patients' tissues including fibroblasts.
These interesting patients highlight that the polyol biochemical pathway is highly active during the first trimester of pregnancy. This pathway seems essential for rapidly proliferating tissues, such as embryonic tissues. In addition to the two well established functions, polyols are organic cellular osmolytes and may play an important role in the water homeostasis of the embryo and fetus. Their high concentration in fetal and placental tissues may contribute to the regulation and maintainance of the cell volume by allowing the extension of amniotic and coelomic compartments during the early stages of pregnancy. Clinical features of TALDO deficiency resembles those seen in neonatal hemochromatosis where an alloimmune mechanism has been recently suggested [25].
Screening for TALDO deficiency by analysis of urinary sugar and polyols should be considered in the differential diagnosis of hydrops fetalis and in neonates and children affected with multi-organ involvement and more particularly with chronic liver disease leading to cirrhosis.

Group 3: Disorders involving complex molecules

This group involves cellular organelles and includes diseases that disturb the synthesis or the catabolism of complex molecules. Symptoms are permanent, progressive, independent of intercurrent events and unrelated to food intake. All lysosomal storage disorders, peroxisomal disorders, disorders of intracellular trafficking and processing such as alpha-1-antitrypsin, carbohydrate deficient glycoprotein (CDG) syndrome, and inborn errors of cholesterol synthesis belong to this group. For many years none was treatable. In the last decade however, efficient enzyme replacement therapy has become available for several lysosomal disorders such as Gaucher, Fabry, Hurler, Maroteaux-Lamy, Pompe and Hunter diseases. Other disorders are at any earlier stage of development or are being explored in animal models [26, 27].

Various cell and organ transplantations strategies have been also developed for certain disorders, some of them successful [28-30], but many others are still experimental [31] or under evaluation. Finally, beside gene therapy [32], new therapeutic approaches such as chaperon therapy appear promising but currently remain mostly inaccessible in clinical practice [33-36]. The first successful stem cell gene therapy using a lentiviral vector in two patients with X-linked adrenoleucodistrophy has been recently reported [37].

In this third category affecting complex molecules, two groups of disorders have expanded remarkably: congenital defects of glycosylation and inborn errors of cholesterol synthesis.
Inborn errors of cholesterol synthesis encompass 8 distinct disorders linked to specific enzyme defects in the isoprenoic/cholesterol biosynthetic pathway [38]. Two of these disorders are due to a defect of the enzyme mevalonate kinase and affect the synthesis of all isoprenoids (mevalonic aciduria and hyperimmunoglobulinemia D). Patients with these disorders characteristically present with recurrent episodes of high fever associated with abdominal pain, vomiting and diarrhea, cervical lymphadenopathy, hepatosplenomegaly, arthralgia and skin rash, and may present with additional congenital anomalies. The remaining 6 enzyme defects specifically affect the synthesis of cholesterol and involve four autosomal recessive (Smith-Lemli-Opitz syndrome, desmosterolosis, latosterolosis and Greenberg skeletal dysplasia) and two X-linked dominant inherited syndromes (Conradi-Hunerman and CHILD syndromes). Patients affected with one of these defects present with multiple congenital and morphogenic anomalies including internal organ, skeletal and/or skin abnormalities, and a marked delay in psychomotor development reflecting cholesterol pivotal role in human embryogenesis and development. All these disorders can be screened by plasma sterols analysis by GC-MS, confirmed by enzymatic and molecular studies. No treatment is available at the present time.
Congenital disorders of glycosylation form another very important and complex group of disorders involving the synthesis of either N-glycans or O-glycans [39, 40].

The synthesis of N-glycans proceeds in three stages (*figure 2*): 1) the formation in the cytosol of nucleotide linked sugars (guanosine diphosphate mannose, uridine disphosphate glucose and UDP-N-acetylglucosamine) followed by attachment of N-acetylglucosamine and mannose unit to dolichol phosphate and flipping of the nascent oligosaccharide structure into the endoplasmic reticulum; 2) stepwise assembly in the endoplasmic reticulum by further addition of mannose and glucose; 3) transfer of these precursors onto the nascent protein followed by final processing of the glycan in the Golgi complex. At the present time, twelve CDG type I have been identified (Ia to Il), ten of them involving the nervous system and two restricted to intestine and liver (CDG Ib and Ih). There are also six already described CDG type II (CDG type IIa to IIf), all but one involving the nervous system. Given the importance of N-glycosylation, patients with CDG form a rapidly growing group with a very broad spectrum of clinical manifestations and should be considered a possible diagnosis in any unexplained clinical condition, mostly in multi-organ disease with neurological involvement. Isoelectrofocusing of serum transferrin and western blot analysis of various glycosylated proteins are the screening methods of choice but only allow detecting N-glycosylation disorders associated with sialic acid deficiency. The distinction between type I and type II relies on the serum transferrin isoelectrofocusing patterns. The most frequent CDG type I are CDG Ia (phosphomannomutase II deficiency) with at least 450 patients known worldwide, CDG Ib (phosphomannoisomerase deficiency) with about 30 known patients treatable with mannose [41], and CDG Ic (glucosyltransferase I deficiency) with about 30 patients already identified.

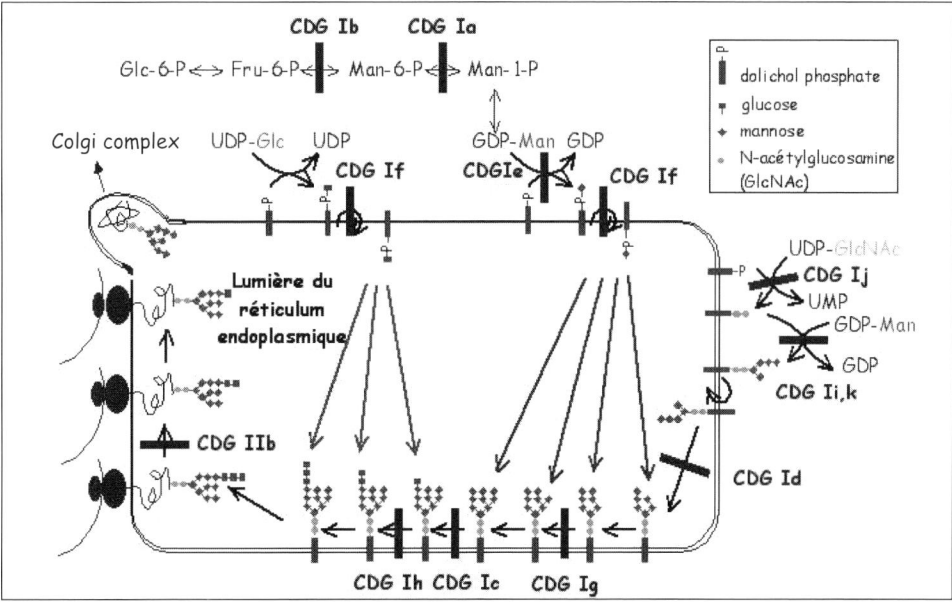

Figure 2. Deficiencies localisation.

Five disorders of O-glycosylation have been already identified: the multiple exostose syndrome and the progeroid variant of Ehlers-Danlos syndrome (both defects in O-glycosylglycan synthesis); the Walker-Warburg syndrome [42] and the muscle-eye-brain disease [43], both secondary to defects in O-mannosylglycan synthesis and presenting with severe neuronal migration disorders with brain and eye dysgenesis, lissencephaly and congenital muscular dystrophy caused by POMT1 and POMGnT1 mutations respectively; finally the familial tumoral calcinosis (defect in O-N-acetylgalactosaminylglycan synthesis). Two newly discovered disorders have also been recently identified: COG7 deficiency [44] and GM3 synthase deficiency [45]. This illustrates the size of this still largely unexplored metabolic field.

Clinical presentation

There are four groups of clinical circumstances in which physicians are faced with the possibility of a metabolic disorder:
– Early symptoms in the antenatal and neonatal period.
– Later-onset acute and recurrent attacks of symptoms such as coma, ataxia, vomiting, and acidosis.
– Chronic and progressive symptoms which can be general (failure to thrive), muscular or neurological (developmental delay, neurological deterioration, psychiatric signs).
– Specific and permanent adverse effects on various organs or systems.

The first two categories often present as treatable emergencies, either in the neonatal period or late in infancy to adulthood. Main chronic or progressive symptoms and signs which raise suspicion of a treatable IEM are mostly nutritional (failure to thrive) and neurological. An important emerging concern is the late presentations in adolescence and adulthood [2].

Newborn screening for inborn errors of metabolism

Newborn screening has opened new perspectives in preventive medicine. Babies with disorders of amino acid, organic acid and fatty acid metabolism are now often detected in the newborn screening laboratory (already available in many European and non European countries) rather than by the clinical metabolic service. Tandem mass spectrometry has revolutionized newborn screening. Early detection provides three possibilities [46]: 1) the disorder may present in the first days of life before any newborn screening result is likely: disorders in this category include neonatal presentations of urea cycle defects, organic acidaemias such as methylmalonic academia, and less commonly almost any of the fatty acid oxidation defects. Detection by newborn screening is unlikely to benefit directly most cases in this category. However, it seems appropriate to include these early presenting disorders in the screening suite as some may have delayed diagnosis and on occasion a diagnosis may never be made, the baby having been thought to have died from sepsis. 2) The disorder may be later presenting and an effective treatment can beneficially alter the natural history: cases in this category include the less severe urea cycle disorders, most aminoacidopathies (such as phenylketonuria, homocystinuria, maple syrup urine disease), some organic acidaemias and most fatty acid oxidation disorder cases. 3) The disorder may be benign or largely so and most cases will have no benefit from early diagnosis. It is hard to know yet which cases will fit into this category. If that was clear, then the disorders could be removed from the screening suite but newborn screening if carefully and sensitively conducted, provides an excellent opportunity for elucidating the natural history of disorders which might or might not fall into this category. What is clear is that mild forms of several disorders will readily be detected by newborn screening but will not need treatment. All these aspects raise many organisational, practical and ethical questions.

References

1. Raine DN. *The Treatment of Inherited Metabolic Disease*. Lancaster: Medical and Technical Publishing Co. Ltd, 1975, 294 p.
2. Saudubray JM, Sedel F, Walter JH. Clinical approach to treatable inborn metabolic diseases: an introduction. *J Inher Metab Dis* 2006; 29: 261-74.
3. Junien C. Impact of diets and nutrients/drugs on early epigenetic programming. *J Inher Metab Dis* 2006; 29: 359-65.
4. Clayton PT. B6-responsive disorders: a model of vitamin-dependency. *J Inher Metab Dis* 2006; 29: 317-26.
5. Hunt AD, Stokes J, McCrory WW, Stroud HH. Pyridoxine dependency: report of a case of intractable convulsions in an infant controlled by pyridoxine. *Pediatrics* 1954; 13: 140-5.
6. Mills PB, Struys E, Jakobs C, et al. Mutations in antiquitin in individuals with pyridoxine-dependent seizures. *Nat Med* 2006; 12: 307-9.
7. Mills PB, Surtees RA, Champion MP, et al. Neonatal epileptic encephalopathy caused by mutations in the PNPO gene encoding pyridox (am) ine 5'-phosphate oxidase. *Hum Mol Genet* 2005; 14: 1077-86.
8. Hoffmann GF, Schmitt B, Windfurh, et al. Pyridoxal 5'-phosphate may be curative in early-onset epileptic encephalopathy. *J Inherit Metab Dis* 2007; 30: 96-9.
9. Mudd SH, Levy HL, Kraus JP. Disorders of transsulfuration. In: Scriver CR, Beaudet AL, Sly WS, Valle D, eds. *The metabolic and molecular bases of inherited disease*, 8th edn. New York: McGraw-Hill, 2001: 2007-56.

10. de Koning TJ. Treatment with amino acids in serine deficiency disorders. *J Inher Metab Dis* 2006; 29: 347-51.
11. Jaeken J, Detheux M, van Maldergem L, et al. 3-Phosphoglycerate dehydrogenase deficiency: an inborn error of serine biosynthesis. *Arch Dis Child* 1996; 74: 542-5.
12. de Koning TJ, Klomp LW, van Oppen AC, et al. Prenatal and early postnatal treatment in 3-phosphoglycerate-dehydrogenase deficiency. *Lancet* 2004; 364: 2158-60.
13. Häberle J, Görg B, Rutsch F, et al. Congenital glutamine deficiency with glutamine synthetase mutations. *N Engl J Med* 2005; 353: 1926-33.
14. Häberle J, Görg B, Toutain A, et al. Inborn error of amino acid synthesis: human glutamine synthetase deficiency. *J Inher Metab Dis* 2006; 29: 352-8.
15. Quinzii C, Naini A, Salviati L, et al. A mutation in para-hydroxybenzoate-polyprenyl transferase (COQ2) causes primary Coenzyme Q10 deficiency. *Am J Hum Genet* 2006; 78: 345-9.
16. Roe CR, Mochel F. Anaplerotic diet therapy in inherited metabolic disease: therapeutic potential. *J Inher Metab Dis* 2006; 29: 332-40.
17. Van Spronsen FJ, Smit GPA, Erwich JJHM. Inherited metabolic diseases and pregnancy. *BJOG: an International Journal of Obstetrics and Gynaecology* 2005; 112: 2-11.
18. Valayannopoulos V, Verhoeven NM, Mention K, et al. Transaldolase deficiency: a new cause of hydrops foetalis and neonatal multiorgan disease. *J Pediatr* 2006; 149: 713-7.
19. Klepper J, Voit T. Facilitated glucose transporter protein type 1 (GLUT1) deficiency syndrome: impaired glucose transport into brain – a review. *Eur J Pediatr* 2002; 161: 295-304.
20. de Vivo DC, Leary L, Wang D. Glucose transporter 1 deficiency syndrome and other glycolytic defects. *J Child Neurol* 2002; 17: 3S15-3S23.
21. Santer R, Schneppenheim R, Dombrowski A, et al. Mutations in GLUT2, the gene for the liver-type glucose transporter, in patients with Fanconi-Bickel syndrome. *Nat Genet* 1997; 17: 324-6.
22. Santer R, Schneppenheim R, Suter D, et al. Fanconi-Bickel syndrome – the original patient and his natural history, historical steps leading to the primary defect, and a review of the literature. *Eur J Pediatr* 1998; 157: 783-97.
23. Huck JH, Verhoeven NM, Struys EA, et al. Ribose-5-phosphate isomerase deficiency: new inborn error in the pentose phosphate pathway associated with a slowly progressive leukoencephalopathy. *Am J Hum Genet* 2004; 74: 745-51.
24. Verhoeven NM, Huck JH, Roos B, et al. Transaldolase deficiency: liver cirrhosis associated with a new inborn error in the pentose phosphate pathway. *Am J Hum Genet* 2001; 68: 1086-92.
25. Whitington PF, Malladi P. Neonatal hemochromatosis: is it an alloimmune disease? *J Pediatr Gastroenterol Nutr* 2005; 40: 544-9.
26. Desnick RJ. Enzyme replacement and enhancement therapies for lysosomal diseases. *J Inher Metab Dis* 2004; 27: 385-410.
27. Wraith JE. Limitations of enzyme replacement therapy: current and future. *J Inher Metab Dis* 2006; 29: 442-7.
28. Sokal EM. Liver transplantation for inborn errors of liver metabolism. *J Inher Metab Dis* 2006; 29: 426-30.
29. Dhawan A, Mitry RR, Hughes RD. Hepatocyte transplantation for liver-based metabolic disorders. *J Inher Metab Dis* 2006; 29: 431-5.
30. Boelens JJ. Trends in haematopoietic cell transplantation for inborn errors of metabolism. *J Inher Metab Dis* 2006; 29: 413-20.
31. Weber A, Mahieu-Caputo D, Hadchouel M, Franco D. Hepatocyte transplantation: studies in preclinical models. *J Inher Metab Dis* 2006; 29: 436-41.
32. Fischer A, Hacein-Bey-Abina S, Cavazzana-Calvo M. Gene therapy of metabolic diseases. *J Inher Metab Dis* 2006; 29: 409-12.
33. Gregersen N. Protein misfolding disorders: pathogenesis and intervention. *J Inher Metab Dis* 2006; 29: 456-70.
34. Aerts JMFG, Hollak CEM, Boot RG, et al. Substrate reduction therapy of glycosphingolipid storage disorders. *J Inher Metab Dis* 2006; 29: 448-55.
35. Suzuki Y. b-galactosidase deficiency: an approach to chaperone therapy. *J Inher Metab Dis* 2006; 29: 471-6.

36. Amaral MD. Therapy through chaperones: sense or antisense? Cystic fibrosis as a model disease. *J Inher Metab Dis* 2006; 29: 477-87.
37. Cartier N, Aubourg P, et al. Successful stem cell gene therapy using a lentiviral vector in 2 XALD patients. *Hum Gen Ther* 2007; 18: 1941 (abstract).
38. Waterham HR, Clayton PT. Disorders of cholesterol synthesis. In: Fernandes J, Saudubray JM, van den Berghe G, Walter J, eds. *Inborn Metabolic Diseases: Diagnosis and Treatment*, 4th edn. Berlin: Springer-Verlag, 2006: 412-420.
39. Jaeken J. Komrower Lecture. Congenital disorders of glycosylation (CDG): it's all in it! *J Inher Metab Dis* 2003; 26: 99-118.
40. Marquardt T, Denecke J. Congenital disorders of glycosylation: review of their molecular bases, clinical presentations and specific therapies. *Eur J Pediatr* 2003; 16: 359-79.
41. Niehues R, Hasilik M, Alton G, et al. Carbohydrate-deficient glycoprotein syndrome type Ib. Phosphomannose isomerase deficiency and mannose therapy. *J Clin Invest* 1998; 101: 1414-20.
42. Beltran-Valero de Bernabé D, Currier S, Steinbrecher A, et al. Mutations in the O-mannosyltransferase gene POMT1 give rise to the severe neuronal migration disorder Walker-Warburg syndrome. *Am J Hum Genet* 2002; 71: 1033-43.
43. Yoshida A, Kobayashi K, Manya H, et al. Muscular dystrophy and neuronal migration disorder caused by mutations in a glycosyltransferase, POMGnT1. *Dev Cell* 2001; 1: 717-24.
44. Spaapen LJ, Bakker JA, van der Meer SB, et al. Clinical and biochemical presentation of siblings with COG-7 deficiency, a lethal multiple O- and N-glycosylation disorder. *J Inher Metab Dis* 2005; 28: 707-714.
45. Simpson MA, Cross H, Proukakis C, et al. Infantile-onset symptomatic epilepsy syndrome caused by a homozygous loss-of-function mutation of GM3 synthase. *Nat Genet* 2004; 36: 1147-8.
46. Wilcken B. Newborn screening for inborn errors of metabolism. In: Fernandes J, Saudubray JM, van den Berghe G, Walter J, eds. *Inborn Metabolic Diseases: Diagnosis and Treatment*, 4th edn. Berlin: Springer-Verlag, 2006: 50-7.

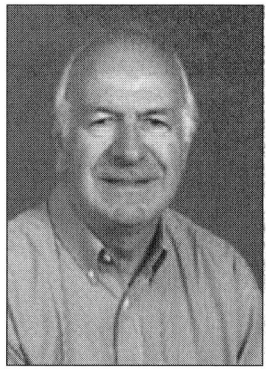

Progress in Paediatric Endocrinology 2001-2006

Martin O. SAVAGE

*Department of Paediatric Endocrinology,
Barts and London School of Medicine, London, United Kingdom*

Introduction

The period of the last five years has seen remarkable progress in several areas of paediatric endocrinology, which have resulted in changes in clinical practice. Important advances relate to three main fields; molecular investigations and the elucidation of key physiological mechanisms, technical advances in patient investigation and progress in therapy. This chapter will give examples of such progress and will concentrate on the fields of growth hormone deficiency and resistance and adreno-cortical deficiency and hyperfunction.

Molecular delineation of physiology and pathophysiology of the growth hormone insulin-like growth factor-I axis

The integrity of the growth hormone (GH) insulin-like growth factor-I (IGF-I) axis is crucial for normal linear growth during childhood and for normal carbohydrate and lipid metabolism during adult life. Detailed molecular investigations of children with growth failure resulted in the identification of novel gene defects which have helped to explain the physiology of this axis. The molecular genetic analysis of DNA from patients and families with severe GH deficiency or action has resulted in some remarkable discoveries.

GH deficiency

The genetic origins of severe or congenital GH deficiency have been investigated in a number of centres. The previous five years saw the identification of defects in the pituitary development transcription factors Pit 1 and PROP 1 and the identification of the first gene defect, namely of *HESX1* in patients with the phenotype of septo-optic dysplasia [1].

The phenotypic spectrum of congenital hypopituitarism was broadened by the description of a new syndrome with associated features of a short rigid cervical spine with limited head rotation and mutations of the homeobox genes *LHX3* and *LHX4* [2, 3]. These defects have broadened the genetic and phenotypic spectrum of paediatric hypopituitarism. The identification of these new molecular defects was performed in the laboratory of Serge Amselem in Créteil, France.

GH resistance

The field of GH resistance became open to molecular investigation following the cloning of the GH receptor (GHR). During the 1980s and 1990s many mutations of the GHR, causing the most severe form of GH resistance, Laron syndrome, were identified and published. These have been recently reviewed [4]. It became clear that the population of GH resistant patients, although small, was heterogeneous [5] (*figure 1*) and a significant proportion of these subjects had normal molecular sequence of the GHR. Consequently the search began for gene defects downstream from the GHR (*figure 2*). Rosenfeld's group made a key contribution to the literature with the identification of mutations in the gene for the post-GHR signalling molecule STAT5b [6, 7]. Affected patients have an interesting phenotype which combines severe short stature and GH resistance with immunological abnormalities related to defective cytokine signalling, which also depends on the integrity of STAT5b. Seven patients have now been reported definitively or in abstract form, suggesting that this genetic defect may be the commonest in GH resistant patients with a normal GHR sequence. The presence of a previously unidentified GHR intronic mutation causing a pseudoexon which may impair GHR dimerization has also been described in patients who were considered to have a normal GHR sequence [8].

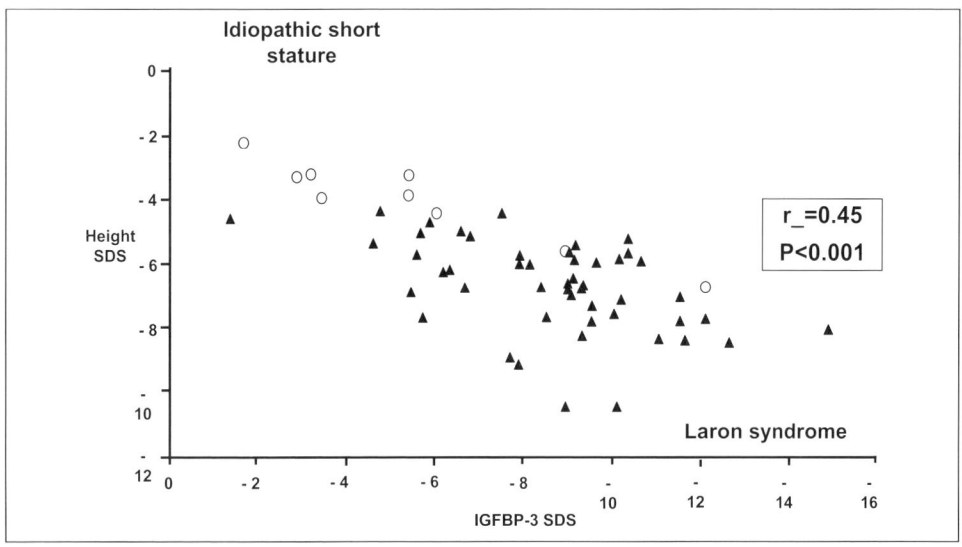

Figure 1. Variation in clinical phenotype from Laron syndrome (triangles) to idiopathic short stature (circles) across the spectrum of 58 patients with GH insensitivity from the European series (Burren *et al.* 2001). IGFBP-3: insulin-like growth factor binding protein-3; SDS: SD score.

More recently another key genetic defect was identified in patients with short stature, namely a mutation in the gene for acid labile subunit (ALS) (*Figure 2*). This defect was first described by Domene *et al.* from Buenos Aires [9]. The phenotype is interesting, because the original patient had only a mild degree of short stature. Endocrine investigations showed extreme GH resistance and IGF-I deficiency with undetectable levels of ALS. It is possible however that the defect causes predominant deficiency of circulating IGF-I, because the ternary complex consisting of IGF-I, IGFBP-3 and ALS cannot be formed. Paracrine IGF-I may therefore be normal and hence linear growth is only slightly affected. A subsequent case of ALS gene mutation has recently been reported [10].

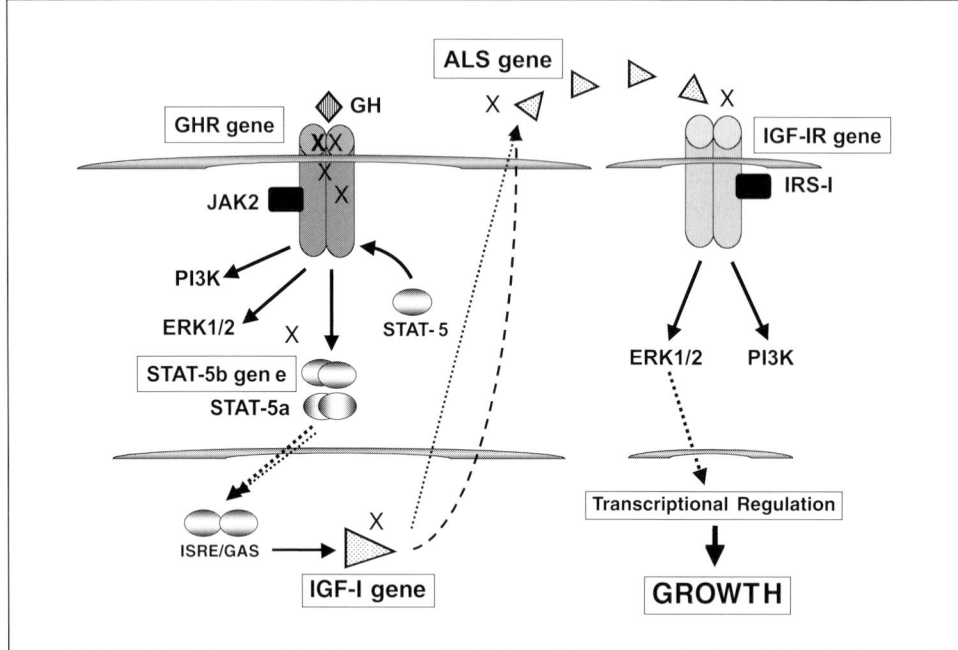

Figure 2. GH receptor and post-GH receptor defects causing GH insensitivity. Sites of gene defects are shown by the X symbol.
This figure is reproduced with kind permission of Dr RG Rosenfeld and Dr V Hwa.

IGF-I and IGF-I receptor gene mutations

Moving further down the GH-IGF-I axis (*Figure 2*), a key publication complimented the original description of an IGF-I gene deletion [11]. The new publication from the group of Jan-Maarten Wit in Leiden, Netherlands confirmed the existence of the original phenotype, by describing an adult patient with severe short stature, microcephaly, deafness, intellectual retardation and insulin resistance [12]. In contrast to the patient described by Woods *et al.* the patient from the Netherlands had elevated serum IGF-I levels but demonstrated lack of IGF-I binding to its receptor. This demonstrated that the mutation in the IGF-I gene had resulted in immuno-assayable IGF-I which was biologically inactive.

One of the key findings from the IGF-I gene mutations patients was the presence of intrauterine growth retardation (IUGR). This finding confirmed that IGF-I production and action are essential for normal fetal growth. It was therefore logical to try to identify cases with mutations in the IGF-I receptor (IGF-IR), a much larger gene, amongst a population of IUGR patients. Such a project was performed by the groups of Chernausek in Cincinatti and Kiess in Leipzig. This collaboration led to the outstanding publication of the first cases with molecular evidence of mutations in the IGF-I receptor gene [13]. The different endocrine and phenotypic features of GHR, post-GHR, IGF-I gene and IGF-IR gene mutations are shown in *table 1*.

Table 1. Comparison between patients with different genetic defects of the GH-IGF-I axis.

Adapted from Chernausek SD, Abuzzahab MJ, Kiess W, Osgood D, Schneidser A, Smith RJ. IGF resistance: The role of the type 1 IGF receptor. *In: Deciphering growth.* (eds) Carel J-C, Kelly PA, Christen Y. Springer-Verlag, Berlin, Heidelberg, New York 2005, 121-30.

	GH Receptor Deficiency*	GH Post-Receptor (Stat 5b)	IGF-I gene Defect	IGF-I Receptor Deficiency
GH secretion	Increased	Increased	Increased	Varied
Serum IGF-I	Very low	Very low	Absent or increased if biologically inactive	Normal to Increased
Serum IGF-II	Low	n/a	Normal	Normal
Prenatal growth	Near normal	Near normal	IUGR	IUGR
Postnatal growth	Very slow	Very slow	Very slow	Very slow
Skeletal material	Very delayed	n/a	Modest delay	Modest delay
CNS	Near normal	n/a	Retarded	Variably abnormal
Hearing	Normal?	n/a	Sensorineural deafness	Normal?
Glycemic status	Hypoglycaemia	n/a	CHO Intolerance	CHO intolerance
Dysmorphic features	Frontal bossing Mid-face hypoplasia	Possible milder phenotype	Yes	Variable
Immunologic status	Clinically normal	Impaired, with frequent infections	Clinically normal	Clinically normal

* GH Rreceptor defect, GH insensitivity due to GH receptor deficiency (Laron syndrome); GH post-Receptor, Stat 5b deficiency (Kofoed et al. 2003); IGF-I defect, deficiency of IGF-I gene (Woods et al. 1996); IGF-I Receptor defect, genetic mutations in type 1 IGF receptor; Abuzzahab et al. 2003).

Treatment of IGF-I deficiency

In the 1980s, following the identification of mutations in the GHR in patients with Laron syndrome, recombinant human IGF-I (rhIGF-I) was synthesized and became available for clinical use. A number of publications demonstrated that therapy with rhIGF-I increased growth in patients with Laron syndrome. However supplies of IGF-I were scarce and many patients remained untreated. During the past five years, two important developments occurred. Firstly a new company, Tercica, was created with the prime aim of manufacturing rhIGF-I for clinical use. Using historical data, Tercica's product was approved by the FDA in 2005 for treatment of so-called severe primary IGF-I deficiency.

Secondly, another company, Insmed, developed a complex which combined rhIGF-I and rhIGFBP-3 in a 1:1 ratio. This complex presents the scientifically logical therapeutic approach of replacing these two peptides which are low or absent in the majority of cases of GH resistance. The IGF-I/IGFBP-3 complex was also approved by the FDA for clinical use. Our group performed the first pharmacokinetic studies with the IGF-I/IGFBP-3 complex in GH resistant patients [14]. The results of these studies were published in early 2006 and are shown in *figure 3*. The results of treatment of GH resistant patients with this complex were presented at the Endocrine Society in 2006 and the definitive publication is eagerly awaited.

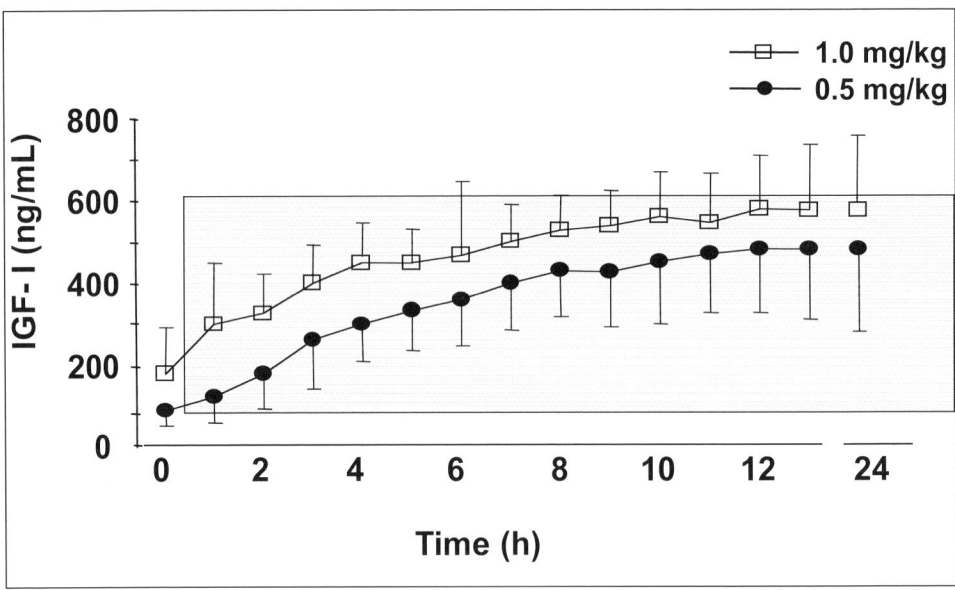

Figure 3. rhIGF-I/rhIGFB-3 pharmacokinetic study. Serum IGF-I levels at baseline and after injection of a single dose of 0.5 mg/kg sc closed symbols or 1.0 mg/kg sc open symbols in 4 patients with GH insensitivity. The shaded area shows the physiological range.
From Camacho-Hübner *et al.* 2006.

Diagnosis and treatment of adrenal disorders

ACTH deficiency

Adrenal insufficiency is a rare problem in paediatrics and a subdivision of this disorder concerns patients with ACTH deficiency. ACTH deficiency may very rarely be isolated associated with mutations of the so-called Tpit gene [15] but is usually associated with other anterior pituitary hormone deficiencies. ACTH deficiency presents a life-threatening situation particularly in infancy and may also occur as anterior pituitary hormone deficiencies evolve during childhood in some genetic or developmental disorders. The assessment of ACTH deficiency in infancy was studied in detail by the group of Dattani in London. Spontaneous cortisol secretion was evaluated and compared with the standard synacthen test (SST). The conclusions were that the SST had only 75% sensitivity and 81% specificity for the diagnosis of ACTH deficiency, when a cortisol value of < 145 nmol/l (-2 SD of the mean of 2 hrly samples for 24 hrs) was taken as the gold standard [16]. Consequently assessment of spontaneous cortisol secretion may be preferable to make this diagnosis.

ACTH resistance

This equally rare disorder is of extreme interest from the molecular point of view. It is traditionally classified into familial glucocorticoid deficiency (FGD) types 1 and 2 [17]. Inactivating mutations of the ACTH receptor (MC2R) account for FGD type 1 and cases without MC2R mutations were hitherto called Type 2. In 2005 the group of Clark in London identified mutations in a new gene in some Type 2 patients [18]. This gene encodes a small single transmembrane domain protein now known as melanocortin 2 receptor accessory protein (MRAP). Several mutations of MRAP have been identified in FGD Type 2 patients. Undoubtedly other genes in this group of disorders will be identified in the coming years.

Cushing's disease

Cushing's disease is a rare disorder in the paediatric age range, but is capable of causing major morbidity. Hence it may present a difficult diagnostic and therapeutic challenge for the paediatric endocrinologist. The state of the art investigation and treatment of paediatric Cushing's disease (CD) was reported from the NIH in 1994 [19]. Since then, investigation techniques have been refined. In our unit in London, in close collaboration with our adult endocrinology colleagues, we have assembled a series of 33 paediatric patients with CD. We noticed that in this paediatric series, males were more frequent, which is unusual in the context of adult CD, where there is a strong female predominace. We studied this carefully and demonstrated a clear excess of males, particularly in the prepubertal patients [20] (*figure 4*). The distribution of sexes changes during and after puberty. This had not been previously reported.

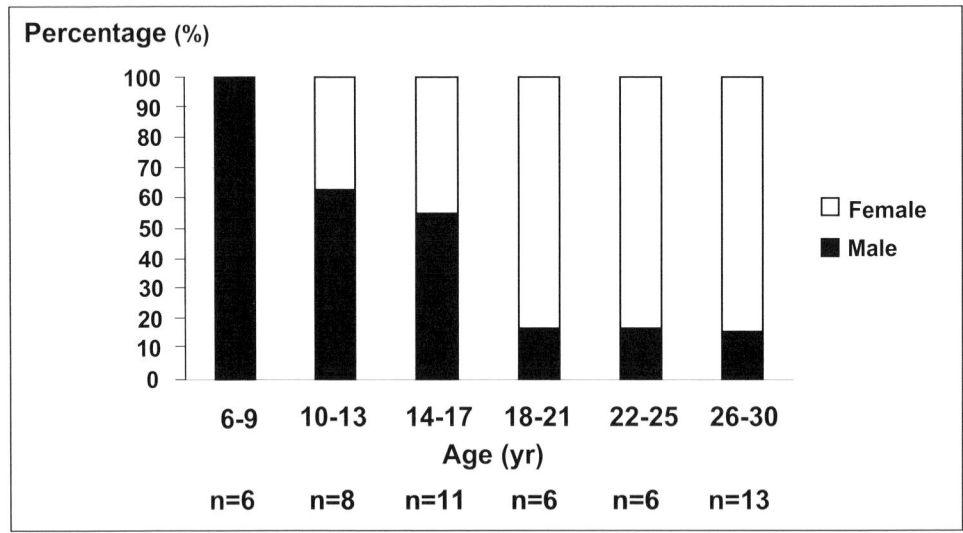

Figure 4. Sex distribution and age of diagnosis in 50 patients with Cushing's disease. From Storr *et al.* 2004.

Children with CD have almost exclusively microadenomas secreting excess ACTH. These may be extremely small and are frequently not visible on MRI scanning of the pituitary. In fact MRI provides a poor prediction of the site of the microadenoma. Transsphenoidal surgery (TSS) is consequently made more difficult by the small size and uncertain location of the tumour. The technique of inferior petrosal sinus catheterisation with sampling for ACTH (IPSS) is well established in adult practice, but although reported by the NIH group in children, has been little studied. We have now performed IPSS in 23 children aged 6 to 17 years and we analysed our results in relation to cure by TSS. Our analysis [21] showed that IPSS provided clear evidence of lateralisation of ACTH secretion in 19/23 patients (83%) and was linked to a high cure rate from TSS of 77% (*figure 5*). We also demonstrated that patients not cured by TSS, respond extremely well to pituitary radiotherapy [22].

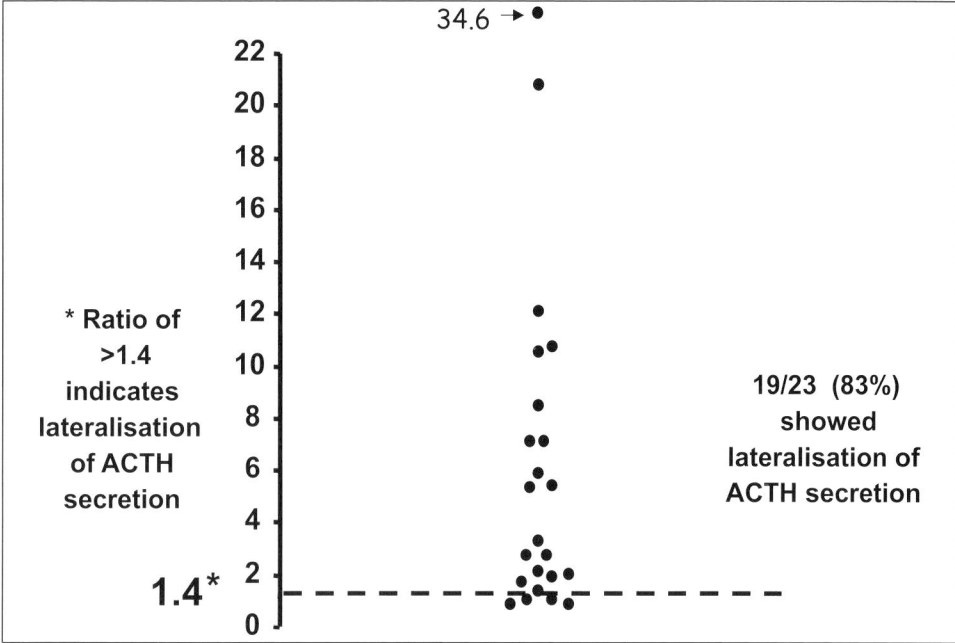

Figure 5. Ratios of ACTH concentrations between inferior petrosal sinuses (IPS) showing lateralization of ACTH secretion during bilateral IPS sampling in 23 paediatric patients with Cushing's disease aged 6 to 17 years.

There are many important advances during 2001-2005 which have not been described in this chapter. Some notable advances in investigation techniques and therapeutic modalities in the field of growth and adrenal disorders have been summarised. They are examples of the directions in which progress in paediatric endocrinology is going. It can be argued that molecular genetics is not making an unequivocal impact on clinical management, however there is no doubt that it has become a vital tool in the assessment of pathophysiological mechanisms and hence the clarification of the origins of disease.

Techniques in the investigation of children, notably in investigative radiology are becoming more and more sophisticated. IPSS is just one example of this. Hopefully the years 2006-2010 will see the continuation of these areas of progress and thereby provide evidence of improved care of children with endocrine diseases.

References

1. Dattani MT, Martinez-Barbera JP, Thomas PQ, et al. Mutations in the homeobox gene HESX1/Hesx1 associated with septo-optic dysplasia in human and mouse *Nat Genet* 1998; 19: 125-33.

2. Netchine I, Sobrier ML, Krude H, et al. Mutations in LHX3 result in a new syndrome revealed by combined pituitary hormone deficiency. Nat Genet 2000; 25: 182-6.
3. Machinis K, Amselem S. Functional relationship between LHX4 and POU1F1 in light of the LHX4 mutation identified in patients with pituitary defects. J Clin Endocrinol Metab 2005; 90: 5456-62.
4. Savage MO, Attie KM, David A, et al. Endocrine assessment, molecular characterization and treatment of growth hormone insensitivity disorders. Nat Clin Pract End & Metab 2006; 2: 395-407.
5. Burren CP, Woods KA, Rose SJ, et al. Clinical and endocrine characteristics in atypical and classical growth hormone insensitivity syndrome. Horm Res 2001; 55: 125-30.
6. Kofoed EM, Hwa V, Little B, et al. Growth hormone insensitivity associated with a STAT5b mutation. N Engl J Med 2003; 349: 1139-47.
7. Hwa V, Little B, Adiyaman P, et al. Severe growth hormone insensitivity resulting from total absence of signal transducer and activator of transcription 5b. J Clin Endocrinol Metab 2005; 90: 4260-6.
8. Metherell LA, Akker SA, Munroe PB, et al. Pseudoexon activation as a novel mechanism for disease resulting in atypical growth hormone insensitivity. Am J Hum Genet 2001; 69: 641-4.
9. Domene HM, Bengolea SV, Martinez AS, et al. Deficiency of the circulating insulin-like growth factor system associated with inactivation of the acid-labile subunit gene. N Engl J Med 2004; 350: 570-7.
10. Hwa V, Haeusler G, Pratt KL, et al. Total absence of functional acid labile subunit, resulting in severe insulin-like growth factor deficiency and moderate growth failure. J Clin Endocrinol Metab 2006; 91: 1826-31.
12. Walenkamp MJ, Karperien M, Pereira AM, et al. Homozygous and heterozygous expression of a novel insulin-like growth factor-I mutation. J Clin Endocrinol Metab. 2005; 90: 2855-64.
13. Abuzzahab MJ, Schneider A, Goddard A, et al. for the Intrauterine Growth Retardation (IUGR) Study Group. IGF-I receptor mutations resulting in intrauterine and postnatal growth retardation. N Engl J Med 2003; 349: 2211-22.
14. Camacho-Hübner C, Storr HL, Miraki-Moud F, et al. Recombinant human insulin-like growth factor (IGF)-I/IGF-binding protein-3 complex administered to patients with growth hormone insensitivity syndrome. J Clin Endocrinol Metab 2006; 91: 1246-53.
15. Vallette-Kasic S, Figarella-Branger D, Grino M, et al. Differential regulation of proopiomelanocortin and pituitary-restricted transcription factor (TPIT), a new marker of normal and adenomatous human corticotrophs. J Clin Endocrinol Metab 2003; 88: 3050-6.
16. Mehta A, Hindmarsh PC, Dattani MT. An update on the biochemical diagnosis of congenital ACTH insufficiency. Clin Endocrinol 2005; 62: 307-14.
17. Clark AJL, Weber A Adrenocorticotropin insensitivity syndromes Endoc Rev 1998; 19: 828-43.
18. Metherell LA, Chapple JP, Cooray S, et al. Mutations in MRAP, encoding a new interacting partner of the ACTH receptor, cause familial glucocorticoid deficiency type 2. Nat Genet 2005; 37: 166-70.
19. Magiakou MA, Mastorakos G, Oldfield EH, et al. Cushing's syndrome in children and adolescents. Presentation, diagnosis, and therapy. New Eng J Med 1994; 331: 629-36.
20. Storr HL, Isidori AM, Monson JP, et al. Pre-pubertal Cushing's disease is more common in males, but there is no increase in severity at diagnosis. J Clin Endocrinol Metab 2004; 89: 3818-20.
21. Storr HL, Afshar F, Matson M, et al. Factors influencing cure by transsphenoidal selective treatment of pediatric Cushing's disease. Eur J Endocrinol 2005; 152: 825-33.
22. Storr HL, Plowman PN, Carroll PV, et al. Clinical and endocrine responses to pituitary radiotherapy in pediatric Cushing's disease: an effective second line treatment. J Clin Endocrinol Metab 2003; 88: 34-7.
22. Woods KA, Camacho-Hübner C, Savage MO, Clark AJL. Intrauterine Growth Retardation and Post-Natal Growth Failure Associated with Deletion of the Insulin-Like Growth Factor-I Gene. New Eng J Med 1996; 355: 1363-7.

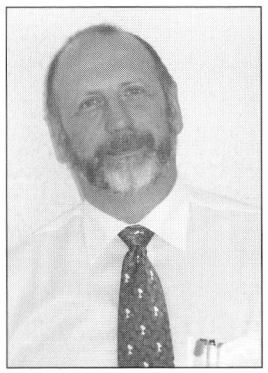

Nutrition in Children: from Calories to Function

Yvan VANDENPLAS[1], Silvia SALVATORE[2], Bruno HAUSER[1], Jean de SCHEPPER[1]

[1] Universitair Ziekenhuis Brussels Kinderen, Brussels, Belgium
[2] Clinica Pediatrica di Varese, Università dell'Insubria, Varese, Italy

Introduction

Nutrition has undergone a major evolution in recent years. For centuries, nutrition was not only considered mainly necessary for survival, but also required for proper growth and development of children. In the developing world, nutrition is still mainly a problem of quantity, whereas in the developed world, interest is focused on quality. In this chapter, characteristics related to the quality of feeding are discussed. The selection of topics is arbitrary, but intended to illustrate the multiple aspects of recent evolution of nutrition: nutri-therapeutics. As a consequence, legislation regarding claims and labelling has become extremely important. The review is far from complete: important areas such as increasing obesity, the metabolic syndrome, anti-oxidants, free radicals, and many other aspects are not discussed.

Gastro-intestinal infection

Worldwide, acute and chronic gastro-intestinal infections still have a major impact on childhood mortality and morbidity. Rotavirus, enteropathogenic *Escherichia coli* (*E. Coli*), salmonella, *Giardia lamblia* and cryptosporidiosis are pathogens more frequently responsible for persisting small bowel damage with increased severity in cases of inadequate initial nutrition and realimentation. Many well-designed studies have tested the efficacy of improved oral rehydration solution (ORS), evaluating the addition of glycine, alanine, glutamine, oligosaccharides or the use of rice versus glucose as carbohydrate. To date, the least one can conclude is that the outcome of these trials is non-conclusive and that results with "classic" ORS are equally good. An exception may be the addition of zinc to ORS. Indeed, different studies show not only a shortening of diarrhoea duration, but also a significant decrease in mortality, even in HIV-positive individuals [1]. Zinc reduces ion secretion and nitric oxide synthesis, improves appetite, absorption, regeneration enterocytes, restoration of enteric enzymes, and humoral and cellular immunity. Zinc also reduces stool output, persistence of diarrhoea episodes and fluid requirement due to its anti-oxidant effects and effects on growth through GH and IGF-1 [2]. Optimal nutritional rehabilitation is consequently considered as the cornerstone of management of (persisting) diarrhoea. Malnutrition not only increases the severity of a gastro-intestinal infection due to an impaired immunological response but also impairs the recovery of damaged mucosa with secondary intestinal and pancreatic enzymatic reduction.

Severe infections increase mucosal permeability and induce local expression of co-stimulatory molecules allowing antigen penetration in the mucosa, T-cell activation and possible disruption of oral tolerance. In the past decades, rapid realimentation in acute gastroenteritis has reduced the incidence of the postenteritis syndrome characterized by food intolerance and persistent diarrhoea. Complex carbohydrates, probiotics and prebiotics such as maize, green banana fibres and pectin have been hypothesized to enhance epithelial gut repair and absorption. L-glutamine, the "fuel" for the intestine, nucleotides, causing proliferation of enterocytes, growth factor(s) with trophic effects on the intestinal mucosa. Bovine colostrum and bovine serum concentrate have also been evaluated, with no evidence of any substantial benefit.

Probiotics, such as some specific lactobacilli (e.g. *Lactobacillus casei* DN-114 001, *Lactobacillus plantarum* 299v) or yeast (*Saccharomyces boulardii*) reduce the invasiveness of intestinal pathogens and beneficially affect the increased intestinal permeability caused by selected bacterial pathogens [3]. However, not all the literature is in agreement: e.g.; administration of *Lactobacillus GG* during 30 days showed no effect on the intestinal integrity of 3 to5-year-old Malawian children with tropical enteropathy.

Enteropathy caused by food hypersensitivity

Coeliac disease

The incidence of coeliac disease (CD) is increasing worldwide, with a prevalence as high as 1 : 80 children. One of the major reasons for the increase in prevalence is improved by serological screening in subjects without overt gastrointestinal complains. However, regional differences are emerging. Wheat, rye and barley are the predominant grains containing gluten peptides, very rich in proline and glutamine and resistant to digestive enzymes, known to cause CD. Variability in the age of symptoms onset, extra-intestinal and autoimmune manifestations, serological positivity, and in severity of histological involvement exists and no clear explanation has emerged despite major advances in identification of toxic peptides, immune cascade and genetic susceptibility. The incidence of CD in mothers giving birth to preterm or dysmature babies was shown to be higher than in a control population (personal data); in other words: undiagnosed CD in pregnant women challenges the outcome of pregnancy, and subsequently the nutritional status of the newborn. Modern histological (Marsh) classification consists of 4 CD types ranging from a normal preinfiltrative stage (Type 0), to infiltrative lesion with increased intraepithelial lymphocytes (Type 1), hyperplastic lesion (Type 2: Type 1 + hyperplastic crypts), destructive lesion (Type 3: Type 2 + variable degree of villous atrophy), and hypoplastic lesion with total villous atrophy and crypt hypoplasia (Type 4). Marsh Type 3 has been subsequently modified into: Type 3a (partial villous atrophy), Type 3b (subtotal villous atrophy) and Type 3c (total villous atrophy). In Marsh Type 1 and Type 2 lesion, positive coeliac antibodies and clinical and serological response to gluten free diet support the diagnosis of CD [4]. After diagnosis of CD, a life-long gluten free diet (GFD) results in disappearance of clinical manifestations, mucosal healing and reduction of CD-related complications. However, the importance of dietetic compliance in asymptomatic patients, the real risk of complications in patients with only subtle mucosal involvement (Marsh Type 1), the individual threshold of gluten sensitivity and the clinical significance of seropositivity in the absence of enteropathy require further clarification. The role of prolonged breast-feeding, timing of introduction and dosing of gluten containing food especially in subjects with a high genetic risk is under evaluation.

Future therapeutic strategies include peptidase supplementation (based on experimental bacterial sources) which cleaves residues next to proline to facilitate proteolysis of immunogenic peptides, transgenic wheat without antigenic peptides, modulation of permeability (by control of the immune cascade and zonulin release) and block of innate and acquired immunity triggered by gluten in coeliac patients. Further efforts are needed to clarify and uniform the definition of GFD, to simplify the labelling of ingredients in food products, to improve and support social life of coeliac patients and to increase early identification of coeliac patients.

Food allergy

Cow's milk protein (CMP), soya, wheat, oats, rice, eggs and fish have all been reported to cause enteropathy in selected children. A 30 kD protein in soya cross-reacts with casein and may favour a concomitant soya and cow's milk hypersensitivity especially in infants with (IgE-negative) CMP enteropathy or enterocolitis. In recent decades an increased number of children have been reported to be sensitised to multiple food antigens, especially (or even) during exclusively breast-feeding, with allergic manifestations early in life due to an impaired development of oral tolerance. In selected infants, acute gastroenteritis increasing permeability and contact of antigens in the lamina propria may provoke sensitisation to dietary antigens.

Chronic diarrhoea, malabsorption, oedema and failure to thrive are the most common clinical manifestations of food related enteropathy. Other gastro-intestinal (abdominal pain, frequent regurgitation or vomiting, constipation, refusal to feed, protein losing enteropathy), dermatological (atopic dermatitis, napkin rash, swelling of the lips or eyes lids), respiratory (runny nose, chronic cough or wheezing, laryngeal oedema), and general (persistent distress, colic) manifestations may be additional features. In many patients, the non-gastrointestinal manifestations are predominant. Especially regarding CMP, most children will tolerate the offending allergen after the age of 1 year although food enteropathy may persist longer in a minority of them.

In food allergy, duodenal, ileal and colonic lymphonodular hyperplasia may be detected as a consequence of immune activation. Histological abnormalities are variable: from total to patchy or even absent villous atrophy, mild to moderately increased intraepithelial CD8 cells, lymphoid follicles, activated lamina propria CD4 cells (with increased IFN-γ ± IL-4 or TNF-α) and decreased regulatory cytokines (especially TGF-β) [5].

In contrast to coeliac disease, enteropathy caused by food allergy presents a thin mucosa, a prominent patchy distribution, only moderate crypt hyperplasia and less intraepithelial lymphocyte infiltration. The infiltration of eosinophils and mast cells is frequent and related to antigen-induced dysmotility and enteric neural dysfunction. The mucosal lesions may cause reduction in brush border disaccharidase expression and secondary exocrine pancreatic impairment, caused by decreased duodenal cholecystokinin production, with mild-to-moderate steatorrhoea and reduced faecal elastase.

As food related enteropathy is mostly cellular mediated, total and specific serum IgE and skin prick tests are often negative. PATCH tests seem to be a promising diagnostic tool for T-cell (late) response to dietary antigen. Faecal calprotectin has been recently proposed as a (unspecific) non-invasive marker of enteropathy.

Mechanisms inducing oral tolerance are, in general, not complete at birth but develop postnatally, mainly in response or intimate relation to the gut flora and to activation of specific Toll-like receptors on regulatory T cells. The key role of the luminal bacteria is highlighted by the impaired tolerance in germfree mice, the different intestinal flora in populations that will develop atopy, the immune-modulatory properties of specific probiotics and by the promising results of interventional studies. Even before the appearance of symptoms, allergic infants have shown a significant higher prevalence of clostridia, coliforms and *Staphylococcus aureus* versus *Lactobacilli* and *Bifidobacteria* (e.g. bifidum dietary supplement). Manipulation of the gut flora as early as in the first days or months of life may have an influence via microenvironment modification and competition subsequent colonization and expression of regulatory cytokines. Specific probiotics including *Lactobacillus* GG (LGG) may induce anti-inflammatory IL-10 and TGF-β and possibly exert a tolerogenic effect before sensitisation occurs. According to 2 trials using supplementation of LGG and *E. Coli* in the perinatal period, in particular non-IgE-mediated allergies are reduced. Maternal supplementation with LGG during pregnancy and 6 months after delivery increases the concentration of TGF-β in the breast milk of at-risk mothers and confer protection against atopy.

Supplementation of a cow milk based formula with prebiotics has the ability to manipulate the intestinal flora with a bifidogenic effect, and a beneficial prospective effect on cow's milk allergy has been recently suggested with prebiotic supplementation.

Prenatal prevention is complex and multifactorial and dietetic intervention during pregnancy is not currently substantiated by scientific evidence [6]. Postnatally, dietetic prevention is currently recommended in high-risk infants only and is based on promotion of breast-feeding (with no conclusive evidence for inconsistently proposed exclusion of peanuts and nuts), hypoallergenic formulas for bottle-fed infants and introduction of solid foods after at least 4, by preference 6, months. Compared to extensive hydrolysate formulas (eHFs), partial hydrolysed formulas offer economical and taste advantages and a theoretical benefit of greater ability to induce oral tolerance to cow's milk protein (CMP) as they still have enough residual allergenicity to induce tolerance but to low allergenicity to induce allergic reactions.

To date, for the treatment of food allergies, guidelines worldwide recommend exclusion of the causative antigen. For the infant who sensitises while being breast-fed, maternal exclusion of the more relevant antigens (cow milk protein, egg's white, (pea) nut) is supported. Infants with cow's milk protein allergy (CMPA) without enteropathy are fed an extensive hydrolysate (eHF), whereas infants with CMPA-enteropathy need a semi-elemental diet (SED). Currently, there is no consensus regarding the optimal management of cow's milk protein allergy. Much debate is on going regarding a "step-up" versus a "step-down" approach. At this moment, the "step-up" approach is mostly endorsed (meaning that allergic children are in first line treated with an eHF and an amino-acid based formula (AAF) is proposed for those infants refusing to drink eHF or SED or those non-responding to the elimination diet. However, one might consider as well to start with an AAF, and challenge with an eHF once the infant is symptom free. The reason for the debate is mainly socioeconomic, and related to the cost of AAF. Infants and children with multiple food allergies have often more severe features with possible reactions even to the small quantity of antigens (like the ones present in breast milk), unresponsiveness to eHFs, and late acquisition of tolerance. The maintenance of a nutritionally adequate diet is not easy especially in cases of compromised absorption or multiple allergies but is mandatory for each child. Major advantages derived by manufacturers continuous efforts to offer new formulas with improved hydrolysation, amino-acid profile, additional beneficial components such as prebiotics, probiotics, nucleotides, MCT and long chain polyunsaturated fatty acids, and last but not least cost and taste. In high risk infants who are unable to be completely breastfed, there is evidence that prolonged feeding with a hydrolysed compared to a cow's milk formula reduces infant and childhood allergy and infant CMA [7]. Three trials have compared prolonged feeding with an extensive to a partially hydrolysed formula and reported no significant difference in allergy incidence in infancy.

Eosinophilic gastroenteropathy and oesophagitis

Eosinophilic enteropathies are (in Europe) rare conditions with eosinophil-rich inflammation in the absence of known causes for eosinophilia (e.g. drug reactions, parasitic infections and malignancy) that may affect part or all of the gut (oesophagus, stomach, small and large bowel) and different layers of the intestine, such as the mucosa, submucosa, muscular layer or serosa. Pathophysiology and therapeutic approach differ according to the type of eosinophilic gastroenteropathy. The disease often has patchy involvement and normal macroscopic appearance, necessitating the analysis of multiple biopsy specimens and quantification of eosinophil infiltration from each intestinal segment. Clinical manifestations are variable, including vomiting, dysphagia, abdominal pain, diarrhoea, bloody stools, iron-deficiency anaemia, malabsorption, protein-losing enteropathy, failure to thrive, obstructive symptoms, and even ascites in the serosal form. A trial of specific food antigen and aeroallergen avoidance is often indicated and in selected cases, an elemental formula is required. Glucocorticoids (systemic or topical) have also showed beneficial results, especially in eosinophilic oesophagitis. Other treatments, such as cromoglycate, montelukast, ketotifen, suplatast tosilate, mycophenolate mofetil, "alternative Chinese medicines," anti-IL-5, the tyrosine kinase inhibitor imatinib mesylate, CCR3 antagonists, and IL-4/IL-13 inhibitors have all been attempted to decrease eosinophilic infiltration but without clear evidence [8]. The primary pathogenic role of eosinophils and of food and inhalant allergens remains to be established. Eosinophilc oesophagitis is a specific entity, different from eosinophilic gastroenteropathy. The incidence of eosinophilic oesophagitis has major regional differences.

Crohn's disease

Crohn's disease may affect any part of the gut (most commonly the ileum and colon) with patchy mucosal ulceration and transmural inflammation due to excess (Th1 and macrophages) immune activation, increased free radicals and overexpression of matrix metalloproteinasis. CD results from a complex interaction among immune, genetic and environmental factors producing a dysregulated immune response to the gut flora. Tolerance to autologous flora appears to be lost and thus luminal "content" represents a persisting driving factor of cell mediated inflammatory process further stimulated by a possible defective response to (selected?) pathogens. The concept that the enteric flora is of profound importance in the development of Crohn's is supported by the absence of disease in germ-free conditions, by the recognition that a specific disease-associated gene such as Nod-2 encodes an intracellular molecule important in the inflammatory response to bacterial peptidoglycans and by the production of IFN-γ inducted in these patients by extracts of their own commensal flora. Furthermore, recent studies showed reduced defensin expression, defective activation of NF-κβ and IL-8 secretion and enhanced IL-12 production (due to a failed inhibition of TLR2 signalling). Selected probiotics could, in theory, restore luminal balance and exert regulatory or anti-inflammatory effects. However, a recent randomised, placebo-controlled trial of LGG supplements in add-on to standard therapy did not prolong remission in 39 children with CD [9]. Thus, interaction between the luminal antigens (from dietary products and microorganisms) and the immune system is crucial and beneficial manipulation of diet and selected probiotic supplementation is intriguing. Many diet trials (i.e. with fibres or carbohydrate restriction or polyunsaturated fatty acid (PUFA) supplementation) have been attempted without significant benefit. The efficacy of polymeric solutions is identical to that of semi-elemental or elemental solutions [10]. Enteral nutrition (EN) with polymeric formula has a proven therapeutic effect for inducing (clinical and histological) remission in paediatric CD. It not only improves weight gain, but also reverses growth failure and nutrient deficiencies. Prolonged nocturnal EN is of great interest for treatment of growth retardation, delay of sexual maturation, in steroid-dependent or refractory CD [11]. Height velocity standard deviation scores were significantly increased in enteral feeding groups compared with corticosteroid groups. Exclusive enteral nutrition (EN) is an alternative to corticosteroids for the treatment of acute flare-up of CD, especially in cases of malnutrition. Some progress has been made in the understanding of the mechanisms by which EN exerts its beneficial influence in CD. Nutritional restitution, modulation of enteric flora and inflammatory cytokines and alteration of the expression of specific genes (with immune effects) within the epithelium have all been considered. A recent report pointed out that the efficacy of EN is significantly dependent on ileal involvement. A profound modification of the faecal microflora after EN (Modulen IBD, Nestlé®) has been demonstrated although the mechanisms of interaction between the formula used and the gut flora still need to be clarified. Modulen IBD has been specially developed for CD and contributes to macroscopic and histological mucosal healing by decreasing mucosal proinflammatory cytokines (IL-1 mRNA in colon and ileum; IL-8 mRNA in the colon; IF-γ mRNA in the ileum) and increasing regulatory cytokine TGF-β mRNA in ileum. In order to increase efficacy, enteral nutrition with a liquid formula should be total: in 50 children with a paediatric CD activity index of more than 20, total enteral nutrition during 6 weeks was almost three times more effective than partial enteral nutrition (50% enteral feeding and unrestricted diet). Total EN decreased diarrhoea, as well as platelets, sedimentation rate, and increased haemoglobin and albumin. Total EN suppresses inflammation in active CD, but partial EN does not. Indications of parenteral nutrition are limited to acute flare-up with resistance to medical treatment and/or EN, and contraindications to surgery, occlusion or fistula, short bowel syndrome.

These results indicate that these formulas have been shown to influence the disease process itself, and thus suggest that the clinical remission achieved is a result of a reduction in inflammation, rather than a consequence of some other nutritional effect. Enteral nutrition is effective in active disease and will induce disease remission in most cases avoiding corticosteroid use. The high frequency of relapse means additional immunosuppressive therapies are usually required but nutrition remains a key priority as part of the subsequent management strategy. No diet has been shown to be effective in long-term maintenance of remission. There is an urgent need for large, multi-centre studies of the different treatment options in paediatric Crohn's disease and the importance of standardized measurements of growth, such as height velocity standard deviation scores and height standard deviation scores as outcome measures [12].

Nutrients

Glutamine

Glutamine supplementation has been reported to be safe, and tends to be associated with less infectious morbidity and mortality. However, glutamine-enriched enteral nutrition did not improve feeding tolerance or short-term outcome in very low birth weight infants and the available data from good quality randomized controlled trials suggest that glutamine supplementation does not confer clinically significant benefits for preterm infants [13].

Nucleotides

Nucleotides have a sparing effect on the *de novo* synthesis during rapid growth and during disease, and therefore also optimize the function of rapid dividing tissue, such as gastro-intestinal tract cells. Animal studies have shown that a diet with, in comparison to a diet without, nucleotides enhances gastro-intestinal growth, gastro-intestinal maturation, recovery after injury of the small and/or large bowel, and increases indices of humoral and cellular immunity. A diet with nucleotides resulted in a higher survival rate after injection of the test-animal with pathogens in comparison to a diet without nucleotides. A diet with nucleotides has also been compared in infants to a diet without nucleotides, and resulted in a lower incidence diarrhoea, an increased antibody-titer after *Haemophilus influenzae* type B vaccine, an increased activity of natural killer cells. Dietary nucleotides in neonatal and infant nutrition result in a catch-up growth in infants with a severe intrauterine growth retardation and have a beneficial effect on the gut microflora, incidence of diarrhoea and the immune function [14]. Yau *et al.* randomized 170 normal 1-7 day old infants compared to a group with and without dietary nucleotides (72 mg/L) during 3 months, and organized a 12 month double-blind follow-up. The incidence of diarrhoea was significantly reduced during the first 6 months of life, whereas at the age of one year there was only a trend suggesting benefit. Serum IgA was increased in the nucleotide group. The antibody response to hepatitis B vaccination was not different between both groups. There was no difference in lower respiratory tract infections, but the incidence of upper respiratory tract infection was increased.

However, nucleotide-supplemented formula has not been shown to confer the same benefits as breastfeeding; it cannot be presumed that nucleotides produce the same benefits for infants as human milk. Therefore, nucleotides are considered to be semi-essential nutrients in preterm and newborn infants. Supplementation of formula with nucleotides is regarded as very safe, and addition to formula should be based on cost/benefit ratio. In "at risk" infants, such as preterm and dysmature infants, and those with gut injury, the benefit is considerably more important than in healthy term born infants.

Lipids

An increasing amount of evidence has demonstrated that adequate dietary lipids are extremely important not only for caloric value but also for immune-modulator effects. Lipids may prevent allergic sensitisation by down-regulating inflammatory response (ω-3 but not ω-6 long chain fatty acids) whilst protecting the epithelial barrier, regulate immune function and modify the adherence of microbes to the mucosa thereby contributing to host-microbe interactions. Medium chain (8-12 carbons) fatty acids (MCT) seems to have more strongly anti-viral and anti-bacterial properties (against RSV, HSV, *Haemophilus influenza* and group B *Streptococcus*) than long chain triglycerides. Medium chain triglycerides protect the gut by modulating the immune response to lipopolysaccharides and enhancing the secretory IgA expression [15]. According to a recent Cochrane review, there is no evidence for a difference between MCT and LCT on short term growth, gastro-intestinal intolerance, or necrotizing enterocolitis [16].

Addition of docosahexaenoic acid (22: 6n-3) and arachidonic acid (20: 4n-6) to standard infant formula results in an increase in CD45RO + (memory/antigen primed T cells) and CD4 + cells, improves IL-10 production and reduces IL-2 levels (nn). Similar to nucleotides, extensive discussion is on going regarding the cost/benefit for the addition of long chain polyunsaturated fatty acids to infant formula [17].

Prebiotics in paediatric nutrition

The World Health Organisation recommends exclusive breast-feeding up to the age of 6 months as first choice infant feeding. Cow milk based formula is considered a second choice infant feeding. However, because of the multiple and important differences in composition between human and cow's milk, many industrial adaptations of cow's milk are mandatory to approach the nutritional and functional effects of human milk. Indeed, the "gold standard" is not mother's milk but "the breast-fed baby".

The presence of 10-12 g oligosaccharides (OS) per litre human milk and the absence of OS in cow's milk is one of the striking differences between both. Due to the absence of OS in cow's milk, formula fed infants have a different microbial colonisation: breast-fed babies have a bifidobacteria-predominant flora, whereas formula fed infants have more an adult-like flora. Bifidobacteria were described as an essential part of the gut flora as early as in 1899. The differences in colonisation between cow and breast milk fed babies are most striking in the gastro-intestinal tract, but do exist as well as at the throat level.

The gastro-intestinal tract is sterile at birth. The establishment of the neonatal, infant and adult gastro-intestinal microflora is a gradual, sequential process; in breast-fed babies, the adult-type of flora develops at about 4 years of age. The gastro-intestinal tract is a complex ecosystem, with more than 10^{9-14} bacteria per g faeces, accounting for over 400 different cultivated species. However, it is known that the majority of species cannot be cultivated with the traditional techniques. Today, approximately 10,000 different strains are known to colonize the human gastro-intestinal tract. There are 10-100 times more bacteria in our gastro-intestinal than we have eukaryotic cells. An adult has over 1 kg of flora.

Different clinical trials have evaluated the effect of OS on the development of the intestinal flora. The addition of a specific OS mixture (0.4 – 0.8 g/dl of 90% galacto-oligosaccharides and 10% fructo-oligosaccharides or inulin mixture) to infant formula was shown to result in a gastro-intestinal flora in preterm and term infants close to the flora of breast-fed infants [18]. The diversity of bifidobacteria species is similar to the one in breast-fed infants. These changes are not only found in the faeces, but also in the caecum. A mixture of short and long chain OS stimulates the development of bifidobacteria over the entire colon, and changes the metabolic activity in faeces. Prebiotics are also shown to restore the abnormalities in gastro-intestinal flora induced by antibiotic use. Two trials with oligosaccharides in the treatment of acute gastroenteritis failed to show any benefit.

Many trials have shown normal growth and development with prebiotic-enriched infant formula. The different mechanisms involved in the benefits of prebiotics may include: a decrease of gut pH caused by an increase of lactic acid-producing microflora, direct antagonistic effects on pathogens, competition for binding on receptor sites, improved immune function, increase of immunomodulatory cells, competition nutrients and other growth factors.

The fermentation profile of a formula enriched in prebiotics is closer to that observed in breast-fed infants compared to infants fed a standard infant formula.

Prebiotics in infant formula or cereals decrease the stool consistency in healthy infants [19]. The administration of oligofructose to infants 6-24 months results in a trend towards fewer febrile events and a decrease in gastro-intestinal symptoms.

Several studies have demonstrated that oligofructose and inulin increase calcium absorption. Also magnesium absorption is increased. Cholesterol and triglyceride levels at the age of 6 months are not altered by addition of 0.6 g/100 ml oligosaccharides (90/10% galacto- and fructo-oligosaccharides) in infant formula (personal data).

Differences in the composition of gut flora between infants who will or will not develop atopic dermatitis are present before the symptoms develop [20]. Different studies with probiotics suggest that manipulation of the flora may result in a decrease of atopic manifestations. The addition of prebiotics to infant formula results in a decrease of *Bifidobacteria adolescentis*. Our (unpublished) data suggest a non-significant trend towards a decrease of atopic manifestations at the age of 3-4 years in infants fed during the first 6 months with a prebiotic-enriched infant formula in comparison to standard infant formula.

The addition of oligofructose to cereals results in adequate growth of the children with a reduced incidence of febrile events, antibiotic use and day care absenteeism. The immunological reaction to measles vaccination is stronger in children that have been given prebiotics. Mice that receive a diet enriched with 1, 2.5 and 5% galacto- and fructo-oligosaccharides show a significantly enhanced systemic immune response type TH1 to vaccination. Prebiotics modulate the cellular immunity.

The ESPGHAN Committee on Nutrition concluded, in 2004, that there was no published evidence of clinical benefits, but that side-effects are absent [21]. To date, (probiotic- and) prebiotic-containing infant formulas have been marketed, but as new safety and efficacy data emerge and the regulatory climate becomes more favourable, the number of products is expected to grow rapidly. Oligosaccharides respect the almost sterile stomach, jejunum and ileum and do not stimulate the growth of pathogens. The addition of oligosaccharides to infant formula results in normal development and a similar gastro-intestinal tract flora in breast and formula fed infants. The initial results that were published suggested that this might as well result in a health benefit of formula fed infants, although this factor still requires confirmation. Inulin has been shown to modulate the gastro-intestinal flora composition and to increase absorption of minerals such as calcium and magnesium. In adults, high doses of inulin have been shown to decrease weight and to decrease serum lipid levels.

Probiotics in paediatric nutrition

Not breast-feeding or giving mother's milk is the gold standard, but what is the effect of mother's milk on the infant. The health benefit of fermented food has been known since ancient times, when Plinius the Old recommended the use of fermented milk, in the year AD 76, for the treatment of infectious diarrhoea. Saran et al. [22] showed that fermented milk during 6 months resulted in a significant better weight gain, associated with a reduction of infectious diarrhoea by 50% in Indian children in comparison to normal milk. Probiotic microorganisms are live microorganisms which when administered in adequate amounts confer a health benefit on the host. There is a multitude of foods and food-supplements containing microorganisms. Fermented alimentation is present in almost all traditional cuisines: most frequently fermented milk, but also fermented fish ("ceviche" in South America), coal ("kimchi" in Korea), etc. Food industry uses selected microorganisms, mainly in milk-drinks or yoghurts. Per definition, these microorganisms need to be prepared, preserved and administered in a viable form, and survive the intestinal ecosystem.

The preventive beneficial effect of probiotic-enriched formula in the developed world is less obvious. Saavedra et al. showed approximately 10 years ago that *Streptococcus thermophilus* and *Bifidobacterium bifidum* prevented nosocomial acquired diarrhoea in children that were hospitalized for a long-term in institutions. Although not all studies show a significant decrease in the number of infectious gastroenteritis episodes, some of them do and all trials show some beneficial trend. Not one study suggests side-effects of probiotic-formula given to healthy infants.

Although data showing the effect of prebiotic oligosaccharides on the immune system are more convincing than those on probiotic strains, clinical data on the prevention of infectious gastroenteritis are missing.

Probiotics are one of the best examples of how some aspects of nutrition or nutrients have undergone an evolution into a grey zone where it is not clear what the primary claim should be: nutrient or drug (medication). While most of the probiotic strains are part of foods (yoghurts), others are commercialized in capsules as food supplements whereas others are registered as medication. Studies have shown that manipulation of maternal vaginal and gastro-intestinal flora results in a decrease in severe pathologies development, such as necrotising enterocolitis in the offspring. Moreover, this demonstrates that manipulation of flora is more than just changing microbes. A biotherapeutic agent is a probiotic with a proven therapeutic efficacy, thus medication. The legislation for food-supplements is entirely different from medication legislation. Since biotherapeutics are registered as medication, these products are subject to strict regulation and quality control. Although some of the probiotic food supplements are of good quality, others are not. Unfortunately, the consumer has no clue to distinguish those products with poor from those with good quality. Different analyses of commercialized food supplements have illustrated the poor quality of many of these products. According to Temmerman et al., more than one third of the commercialized food supplements do not contain one viable strain [23]. The majority of the food supplements (73%) and dairy products (64%) tested have more species that are claimed on the label than can be cultured. Only approximately 10% of the products do contain the strains claimed on the label. Therefore, food supplements are not always, in fact, what they claim to be. Strain specificity is of outmost importance.

Effects demonstrated for one strain cannot be extrapolated to other strains, even if they belong to the same species. Some commercialized products are a combination of different strains. Laboratory and clinical testing of product combination is mandatory, since combination of strains may have an antagonistic effect. The following is an example of the importance of clinical evaluation of strains. The *Lactobacillus* (L) *acidophilus* LB strain has been shown to have antibacterial activity against *E. Coli*. However, if the *E. Coli* is present in the gastro-intestinal tract of the host before the *L. acidophilus* LB, as occurs in acute gastroenteritis, its antibacterial activity is strongly reduced because of a non-specific steric hindrance of the receptor sites. As a consequence, only these probiotics can be recommended in therapeutic indications that are registered as drug and/or for which the commercialized product has been extensively evaluated in clinical trials. Both bacterial and non-bacterial probiotic strains do exist. Bacterial biotherapeutic strains are different strains of lactobacilli and bifidobacteria, but to a certain extent also the non-pathogenic *E. Coli* (*E. Coli* Nissle 1917) and some strains of *enterococci* (although relevant transfer of plasmid induced resistance was reported with *enterococci*). The yeast *Saccharomyces boulardii* is the only non-bacterial biotherepeutic strain known.

A substantial number of published reports suggest a health promoting effect of probiotic microorganisms added to infant formula or to cereals (*tables I and II*).

Table I. Prevention of acute gastroenteritis (mainly by addition of probiotics to infant formula).

Author	Probiotic	Country	Age	N° patients	Reduction diarrhoea
Saran	Fermented milk	India	2-5 years	100	yes
Saavedra	Str thermophilus and B lactis	USA	5-24 months	55	yes
Szajewska	L. GG	Poland	1-36 months	81	yes (rotavirus)
Mastretta	L. GG	Italy	1-18 months	220	no
Chouraqui	B. lactis BB12	France	0-8 months	90	no
Thibault	B. breve c50 Str thermophilus 065	France	4-6 months	971	no

Str: Streptococcus; L: Lactobacillus; B: Bifidobacterium

Table 2. Treatment of acute gastroenteritis.

Author	Probiotic	Dose	Duration (days)	Country	Age months	N° pts	Shortening diarrhoea
Isolauri	L. GG	$2 \times 10^{10-11}$ cfu 2x/day	5	Finland	4-45	71	yes
Raza	L. GG	$2 \times 10^{10-11}$ cfu	2	Pakistan	Mean 13	40	more cured day 2
Shornikova	L. GG	5×10^9 cfu/g b. d	5	Karelia (Russia)	1-36	123	yes (rota)
Shornikova	L. reuteri	10^7 or 10^{10} cfu/g	5	Finland	6-36	66	yes (rota)
Guarino	L. GG	3×10^9 CFU 2X/day	6	Italy	3-36	100	yes
Guandalini	LGG	10^{10} cfu/250 ml 2x/day	5	Europe	1-36 m	287	yes
Simakachorn	heat-killed L. acidophilus LB	10^{10} cfu 2x/day	2.5	Thailand	3-24 m	73	yes
Szymanski	mixture 3 L. rhamnosus strains	1.2×10^{10} cfu 2x/day	5	Poland	2-72 months	87	yes (rota)
Costa-Ribeiro	L GG	10^{10} cfu	?	Brazil	0-24 months	124	no
Khanna	L acidophilus	1.5×10^{10} cfu	3	India	6 – 144	98	no
Salazar-Lindo	L. GG	$5 – 10 \, 10^{11}$ cfu	5	Peru	3 – 36	89	no
Sarker	L. paracasei strain ST11	5×10^9 cfu 2x/day	5	Bangladesh	4 – 24	230	no
Shamir	Str. Thermophilus (a), B. lactis (b), L. acidophilus (b), zinc (10 mg) and FOS	6×10^9 cfu (a) and 2×10^9 cfu (b)	5	Israel	6 – 12	65	yes
Cetina-Sauri	S. boulardii	600	4	Mexico	3 – 36	130	yes
Kurugol	S. boulardii	250	5	Turkey	3 – 84	200	yes
Villaruel	S. boulardii	250 (<1 yr) 500 (>1yr)	6	Argentina	3 – 24	100	yes
Billoo	S. boulardii	500 mg	5	Pakistan	2 – 144	100	yes

L. (GG): *Lactobacillus (caseii GG)*; B: *Bifidobacterium*; Str: *Streptococcus*; FOS: *fructo-oligosaccharides*; S. boulardii: *Saccharomyces boulardii*.

The difference is not always significant, and significant outcome variables differ from paper to paper. However, the trend towards "improvement" is constant. Side-effects have not been reported in healthy infants and children.

Nutrition has become more than ingestion of calories. Currently, nutrition is an underestimated valuable tool in the prevention and treatment of different conditions. Clinical research in nutrition is difficult to perform albeit mandatory because of the possible interactions between nutrients. During recent years, interest has mainly been focused on gastro-intestinal flora and its manipulation, and the impact that changes in flora may have on either general well being or specific conditions such as Crohn's disease and food allergy. During the past few years, hydrolysates have been accepted as effective in decreasing cow's milk protein allergy and atopic dermatitis.

References

1. INCLEN. Childnet Zinc Effectiveness for Diarrhea (IC-ZED) Group. *JPGN* 2006; 42: 300-5.
2. Baqui AH, Ahmed T. Diarrhoea and malnutrition in children. *BMJ* 2006; 332: 378.
3. Allen SJ, Okoko B, Martinez E, Gregorio G. Probiotics for treating infectious diarrhoea. *Cochrane Database Syst Rev* 2004; 2: CD003048.
4. Hill ID, Dirks MH, Liptak GS, et al. for the North American Society for Pediatric Gastroenterology, Hepatology and Nutrition. Guideline for the Diagnosis and Treatment of Celiac Disease in Children: Recommendations of the North American Society for Pediatric Gastroenterology, Hepatology and Nutrition. *J Pediatr Gastroenterol Nutr* 2005; 40: 1-19.
5. Pérez-Machado MA, Ashwood P, Thomson MA, et al. Reduced transforming growth factor-Beta1 producing T cells in the duodenal mucosa of children with food allergy. *Eur J Immunol* 2003; 33: 2307-15.
6. Salvatore S, Keymolen K, Hauser B, Vandenplas Y. Intervention during pregnancy and allergic disease in the offspring. *Pediatr Allergy Immunol* 2005; 16: 558-66.
7. Osborn DA, Sinn J. Formulas containing hydrolysed protein for prevention of allergy and food intolerance in infants. *Cochrane Database Syst Rev* 2003; 4: CD003664.
8. Rothenberg ME. Eosinophilic gastrointestinal disorders. *J Allergy Clin Immunol* 2004; 113: 11-28.
9. Bousvaros A, Guandalini S, Baldassano RN, et al. A randomized, double-blind trial of Lactobacillus GG versus placebo in addition to standard maintenance therapy for children with Crohn's disease. *Inflamm Bowel Dis* 2005; 11: 833-9.
10. Comité de Nutrition de la Société Française de Pédiatrie. Nutritional treatment in childhood Crohn's disease. *Arch Pediatr* 2005; 12: 1255-66.
11. Beattie RM. Enteral nutrition as primary therapy in childhood Crohn's disease: control of intestinal inflammation and anabolic response. *J Parenter Enteral Nutr* 2005; 29: S151-5.
12. Newby EA, Sawczenko A, Thomas AG, Wilson D. Interventions for growth failure in childhood Crohn's disease. *Cochrane Database Syst Rev* 2005; 3: CD003873.
13. Tubman TR, Thompson SW, McGuire W. Glutamine supplementation to prevent morbidity and mortality in preterm infants. *Cochrane Database Syst Rev* 2005 2005; 1: CD001457.
14. Yu VY. The role of dietary nucleotides in neonatal and infant nutrition. *J Paediatr Child Health* 2002; 38: 543-9.
15. Kono H, Fujii H, Asakawa M, et al. Medium-chain triglycerides enhance secretory IgA expression in rat intestine after administration of endotoxin. *Am J Physiol Gastrointest Liver Physiol* 2004; 286: G1081-9.

16. Klenoff-Brumberg HL, Genen LH. High versus low medium chain triglyceride content of formula for promoting short term growth of preterm infants. *Cochrane Database Syst Rev* 2003; 1: CD002777.
17. Field CJ, Clandinin MT, Van Aerde JE. Polyunsaturated fatty acids and T-cell function: implications for the neonate. *Lipids* 2001; 36: 1025-32.
18. Bakker-Zierikzee AM, Alles MS, *et al*. Effects of infant formula containing a mixture of galacto- and fructo-oligosaccharides or viable Bifidobacterium animalis on the intestinal microflora during the first 4 months of life. *Br J Nutr* 2005; 94: 783-90.
19. Moore N, Chao C, Yang LP, *et al*. Effects of fructo-oligosaccharide-supplemented infant cereal: a double-blind, randomized trial. *Br J Nutr* 2003; 90: 581-7.
20. Bjorksten B, Sepp E, Julge K, Voor T, Mikelsaar M. Allergy development and the intestinal microflora during the first year of life. *Allergy Clin Immunol* 2001; 108: 516-20.
21. Agostoni C, Axelsson I, Goulet O, *et al*. for the ESPGHAN Committee on Nutrition. Prebiotic oligosaccharides in dietetic products for infants: a commentary by the ESPGHAN Committee on Nutrition. *J Pediatr Gastroenterol Nutr* 2004; 39: 465-73.
22. Saran, S. Use of fermented foods to combat stunting and failure to thrive: background of the study. *Nutrition* 2004, 20: 577-8.
23. Temmerman R, Scheirlinck I, Huys G, Swings J. Culture-independent analysis of probiotic products by denaturing gradient gel electrophoresis. *Appl Environ Microbiol* 2003; 69: 220-6.

Achevé d'imprimer par Corlet, Imprimeur, S.A.
14110 Condé-sur-Noireau
N° d'Imprimeur : 112321 – Dépôt légal : septembre 2008

Imprimé en France